TEN IN TEN
WEIGHT-FREE
WORKOUTS

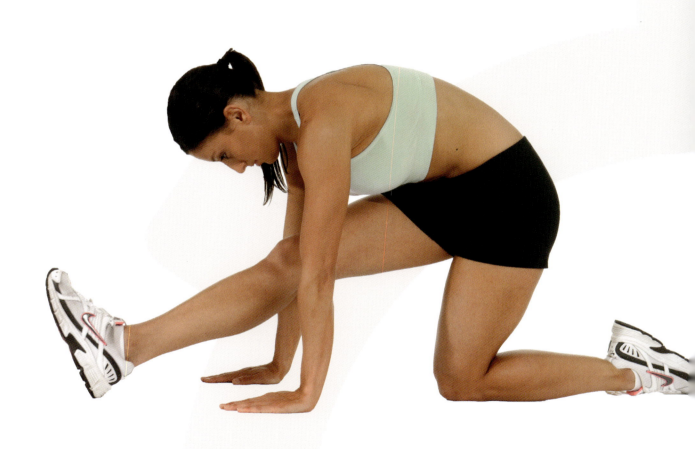

TEN IN TEN
WEIGHT-FREE
WORKOUTS

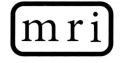

Sean Adams

Published by Moseley Road Inc.

© Moseley Road Inc 2022

Created by Moseley Road Inc.
President: Sean Moore
Production Director: Adam Moore
Layout Designer: Adam Moore
Editor: Finn Moore

Printed in China

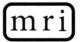

GENERAL DISCLAIMER
The contents of this book are intended to provide useful information to the general
public. All materials, including texts, graphics, and images, are for informational
purposes only and are not a substitute for medical diagnosis, advice, or treatment for
specific medical conditions. All readers should seek expert medical care and consult
their own physicians before commencing any exercise program or for any general
or specific health issues. The author and publishers do not recommend or endorse
specific treatments, procedures, advice, or other information found in this book and
specifically disclaim all responsibility for any and all liability, loss, or risk, personal
or otherwise, which is incurred as a consequence, directly or indirectly, of the use or
application of any of the material in this publication.

Contents

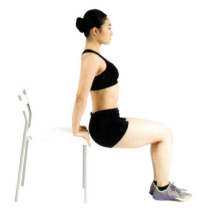

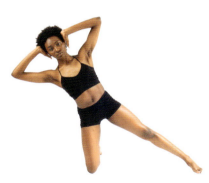

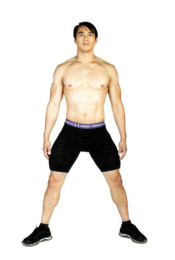

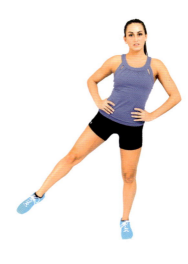

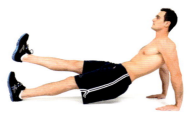

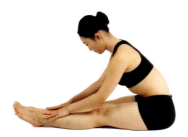

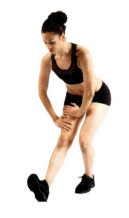

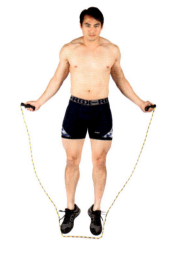

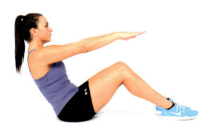

INTRODUCTION

WHY WEIGHT FREE?

Why not? Working out without weights has many advantages, but foremost among them is the fact that you can exercise anywhere, anytime—in your bedroom, in your office, in the park, in front of the TV—all you need is your body and gravity! Exercising weight-free also saves you money—you don't have to buy expensive equipment: no dumbbells, kettlebells, weight racks, resistance machines, and the like; and then there's the fact that you don't need gym membership, and there's no need to drive to the gym three or four days a week, saving on gas too!

That said, there's no need to be purist about it, if you already have weights, or expensive equipment, there's no reason not to use them—this book simply adds variety to your workout routine and gives you options when you are away from home and don't have access to your equipment. Similarly, many people find that the camaraderie of a gym experience is the motivation they need to exercise—this book provides those readers with options while they wait for their preferred equipment to free up.

WHY TEN MINUTES?

The number one excuse for not exercising? "I don't have time". That's fair enough if your workout requires half an hour getting to and from the gym, plus the time spent getting changed, showering, getting dressed—and that's not including the workout! Or maybe the thought of getting the weights out of the closet, or setting up resistance straps just seems like too much effort when you need to get dinner ready in half an hour, or have a Zoom meeting scheduled in twenty minutes, or one of the many other obstacles that life throws in your way. If that sound familiar, this book is for you—it enables you to exercise there and then, whenever the thought occurs to you, and doesn't give you any wriggle room for excuses: we can all find ten minutes! Remove the excuses and you're more likely to exercise.

Maybe ten minutes doesn't seem enough for a meaningful workout? My advice—give it a try! The workouts in this book are devised to add as much variety as possible and after switching through ten exercises in ten minutes, you'll know you've had a workout!

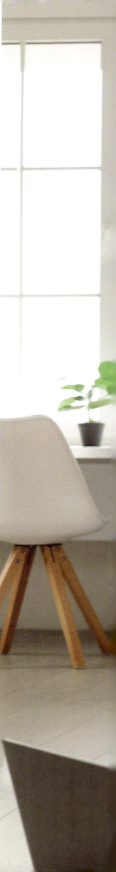

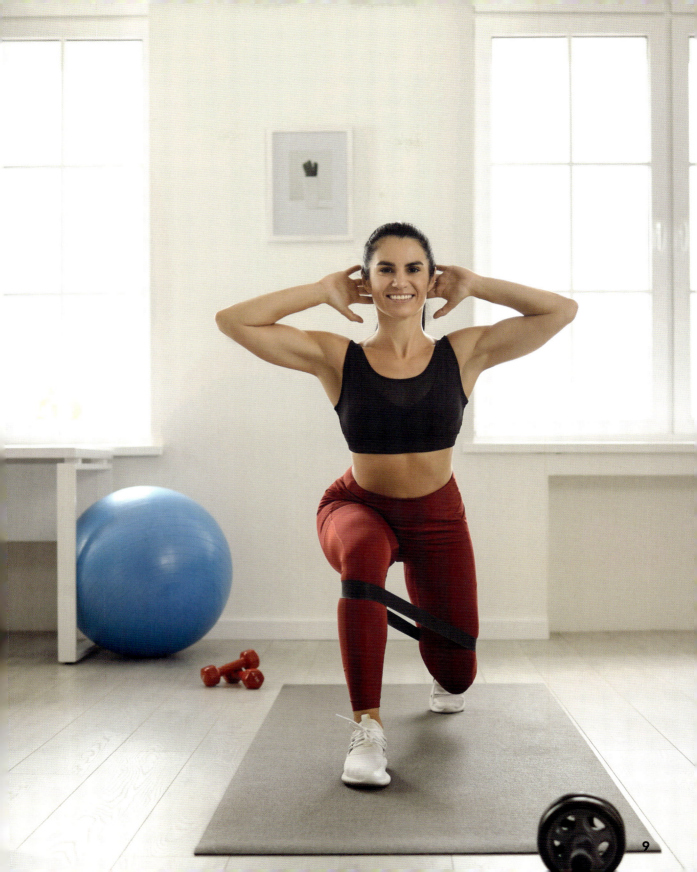

HOW THIS BOOK WORKS

Ten-in-Ten Weight-Free Workouts isis designed to give a perfect workout, whatever your needs or experience levels, and wherever you happen to be, in just ten minutes. Each of the 80+ exercises included in the book has clear step-by-step instructions for how to perform the exercise, plus further instructions of finding the correct form. Every exercise is accompanied by a quick reference list of targeted muscles or body parts, plus detailed anatomical illustrations that add the motivation of knowing exactly which muscles you'll be engaging. The book also includes "modifications" for many exercises—you can make a push-up easier by performing it on your knees for example, or add difficulty by placing your feet on a chair. The Workouts section of the book features only the basic exercises, but feel free to modify them to suit your needs.

Most importantly, the sidebar sets one-minute targets for every exercise for different levels of experience: the Push-Up suggests two sets of eight reps for the beginner, two sets of sixteen for the more experienced, and forty reps for advanced practitioners—but it's important to remember that these are just suggestions: if you can only manage four or five at first, that's fine, you'll get to eight or more eventually. And if you can manage more than two sets of eight in a minute, go for it!

There are ten specially devised Workout routines at the back of this book, a "a basics" workout, one devised for the over-fifties, six body-part workouts, a strengthening routine, and a total body workout.

The Ten-in-Ten premise of the book is aimed at beginner level: ten one-minute exercises adding to a roughly ten-minute workout. As you progress, you will be able to perform more repetitions in a minute, but some of the exercises require holding an exercise rather than repeating it—the Plank, for example—and increasing expertise demands that you hold the position for longer periods: two or three minutes or even longer. The purpose of this book is to encourage you to start exercising, not to limit you to ten minutes!

Finally, the Workouts are also only suggestions—create your own to suit your own requirements or mood—a cardio workout, or a seated workout, or a weight-loss focus, whatever! Just get started, have fun, and get fit!

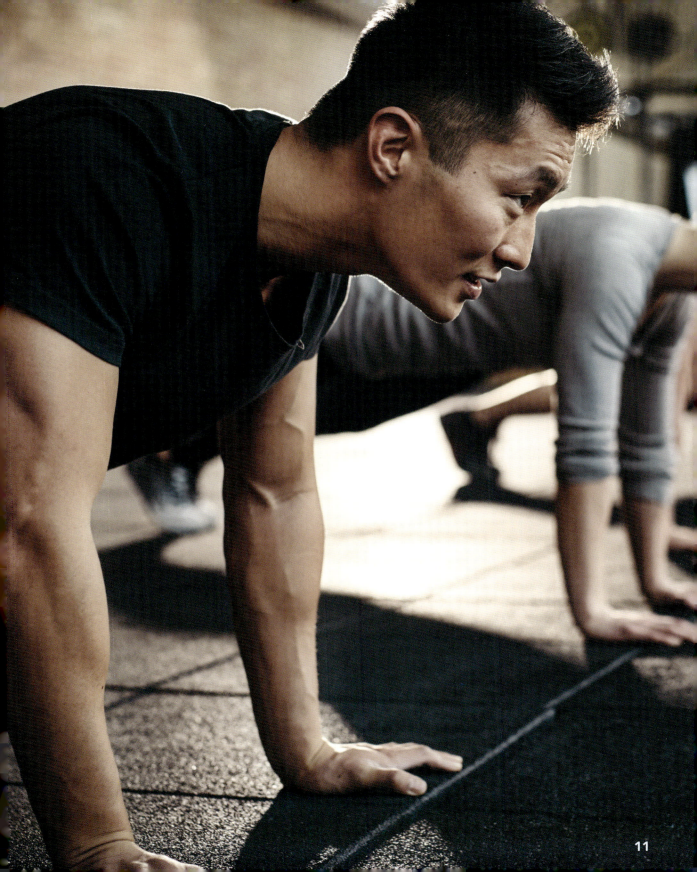

WEIGHT-FREE ANATOMY

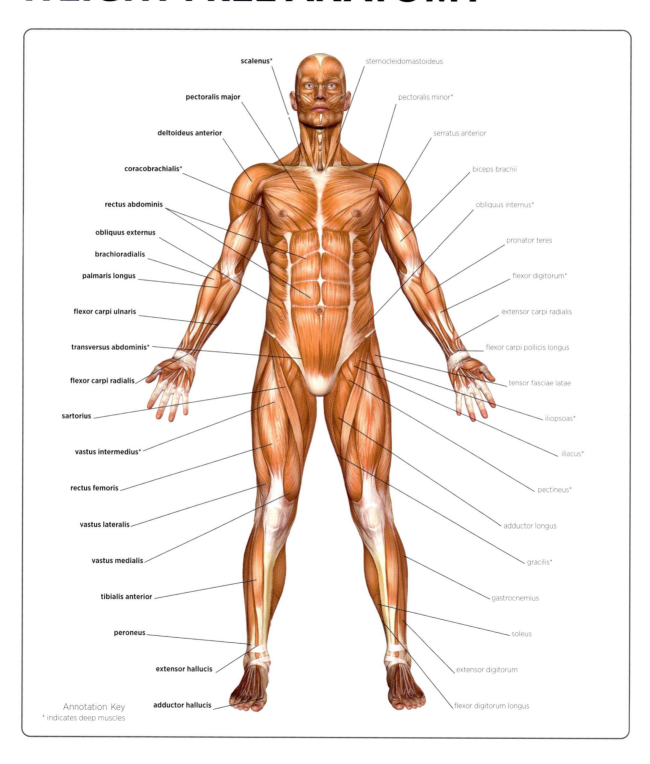

scalenus*

sternocleidomastoideus

pectoralis major

pectoralis minor*

deltoideus anterior

serratus anterior

coracobrachialis*

biceps brachii

rectus abdominis

obliquus internus*

obliquus externus

pronator teres

brachioradialis

flexor digitorum*

palmaris longus

extensor carpi radialis

flexor carpi ulnaris

flexor carpi pollicis longus

transversus abdominis*

tensor fasciae latae

flexor carpi radialis

sartorius

iliopsoas*

vastus intermedius*

iliacus*

rectus femoris

pectineus*

vastus lateralis

adductor longus

vastus medialis

gracilis*

tibialis anterior

gastrocnemius

peroneus

soleus

extensor hallucis

extensor digitorum

adductor hallucis

flexor digitorum longus

Annotation Key
* indicates deep muscles

12

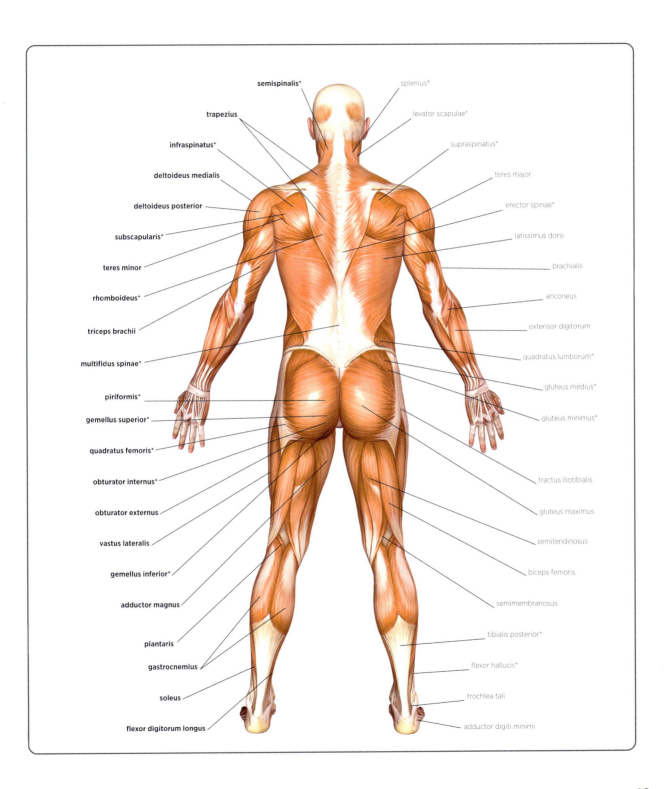

semispinalis*

splenius*

trapezius

levator scapulae*

infraspinatus*

supraspinatus*

deltoideus medialis

teres major

deltoideus posterior

erector spinae*

subscapularis*

latissimus dorsi

teres minor

brachialis

rhomboideus*

anconeus

triceps brachii

extensor digitorum

multifidus spinae*

quadratus lumborum*

piriformis*

gluteus medius*

gemellus superior*

gluteus minimus*

quadratus femoris*

obturator internus*

tractus iliotibialis

obturator externus

gluteus maximus

vastus lateralis

semitendinosus

gemellus inferior*

biceps femoris

adductor magnus

semimembranosus

plantaris

tibialis posterior*

gastrocnemius

flexor hallucis*

soleus

trochlea tali

flexor digitorum longus

adductor digiti minimi

STRETCHING

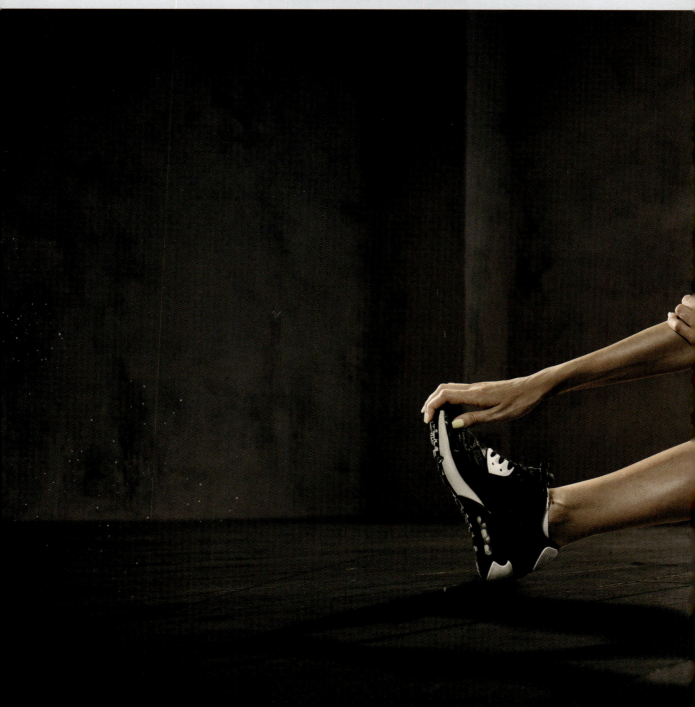

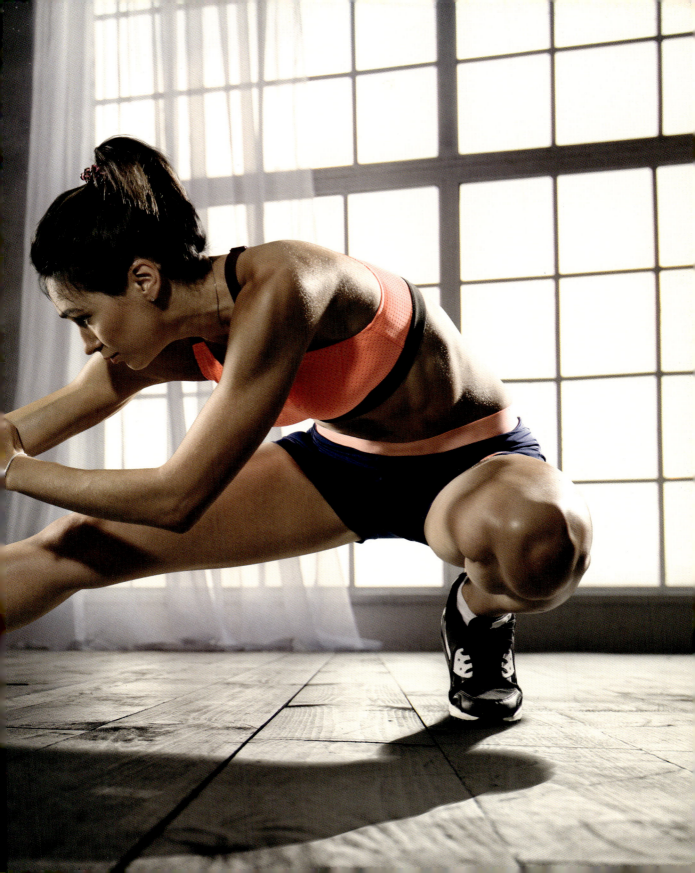

1 MIN TARGETS

BEGINNER
4 x 15 secs

INTERMEDIATE
3 x 20 secs

ADVANCED
2 x 30 secs

BEST FOR

- Abdominals
- Spine
- Shoulders
- Upper back

FIND YOUR FORM

- Keep your elbows slightly bent.
- Tuck your pelvis.
- Avoid hyper-extending either your lower back or elbows.

GOOD MORNING STRETCH

Perform this invigorating stretch first thing in the morning. It will engage your core and lengthen your spine while relieving any tension in your shoulders and upper back that may result from a bad night's sleep.

1 Stand with your legs and feet parallel and shoulder-width apart. Bend your knees very slightly, and tuck your pelvis slightly forward

2 Reach your arms up toward the ceiling, keeping them long and in parallel with your body. Focus your energy on the middle of your palms, which should be facing inward, and turn your gaze upward as you stretch.

3 Hold for the recommended time, release the stretch, and then repeat for the recommended repetitions.

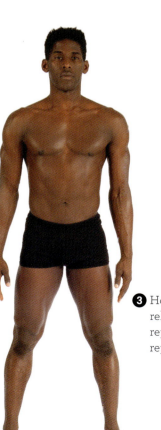

flexor carpi radialis

flexor carpi ulnaris

extensor carpi radialis

extensor carpi ulnaris

palmaris longus

biceps brachii

scalenus*

sternocloidomastoideus

rectus abdominis

obliquus externus*

obliquus internus*

transversus abdominis*

STANDING HAMSTRINGS STRETCH

A simple, effective way to counteract the common problem of tight muscles at the back of the thigh, this stretch should benefit both your calves and your lower back.

❶ Stand with your right leg bent and your left leg extended in front of you with the heel on the floor.

❷ Lean over your left leg, resting both hands above your knee. Place the majority of your body weight on your front heel while feeling the stretch in the back of your thigh.

❸ Hold for the recommended time, release the stretch, and then repeat on the opposite side.

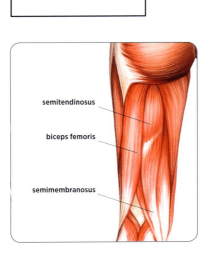

semitendinosus

biceps femoris

semimembranosus

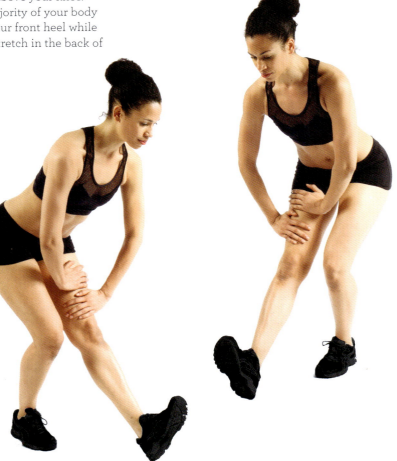

1 MIN TARGETS

BEGINNER

3 x 10 secs per leg

INTERMEDIATE

2 x 15 secs per leg

ADVANCED

2 x 30 secs per leg

BEST FOR

- Core
- Obliques
- Abdominals

FIND YOUR FORM

- Keep your body in a straight line.
- Avoid Raising your leg too high and tipping forward or back

SIDE LYING HIP ADDUCTION

The purpose of this exercise is to strengthen the muscles on the side of your hip. It is a calisthenics and Pilates exercise that primarily targets the glutes and also, to a lesser degree, the obliques, abs, and outer thighs. It gives the upper legs muscle tone.

1 Lie on your left side with your legs extended and your feet stacked one on top of the other. Rest your right arm along your right hip, and use your left arm to support your head.

2 Raise your right leg until you feel your core kick in. Hold for the prescribed time, lower, then switch sides.

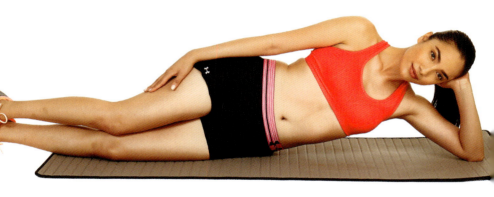

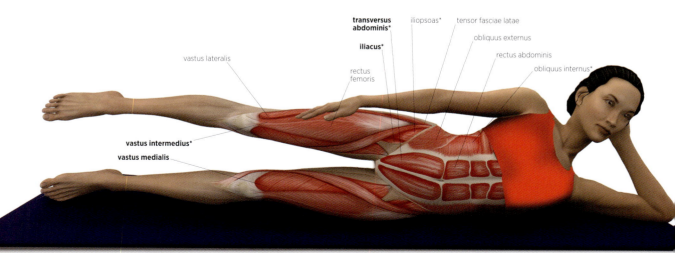

transversus abdominis*

iliopsoas*

tensor fasciae latae

iliacus*

obliquus externus

vastus lateralis

rectus femoris

rectus abdominis

obliquus internus*

vastus intermedius*

vastus medialis

1 MIN TARGETS

BEGINNER
5 reps per leg

INTERMEDIATE
7 reps per leg

ADVANCED
10 reps per leg

BEST FOR

• Calves
• Achilles Tendon

FIND YOUR FORM

• Use a wall or other stable object to balance yourself if necessary.
• Engage all your calf muscles by gently and slowly rolling from your big toe to your pinky toe and back again, shifting your body weight over your toes as you stretch.

HEEL-DROP/TOE-UP STRETCH

The Heel-Drop/Toe-Up Stretch targets the main muscles in your calves—the gastrocnemius and the soleus—and lengthens your Achilles tendon. Stretching the muscles and tendons of your calves should be a consistent part of your lower-body stretching regimen.

1 Stand on an aerobic step, a riser, or a stair with your feet shoulder-width apart and your arms at your sides.

2 Bend your knees very slightly and tuck your pelvis slightly forward. Lift your chest, and press your shoulders downward and back.

3 Place the ball of your right foot on the edge of the step.

4 Drop your right heel down while controlling the amount of weight you put on your right leg to increase or decrease the intensity of the stretch in your calf.

5 Release the stretch, and then repeat on the opposite side.

6 Step down from the riser, and stand with your feet shoulder-width apart. Tuck your pelvis slightly forward. Lift your chest, and press your shoulders downward and back.

7 Position the ball of your right foot on the step.

8 With your knees straight, bring your hips forward to feel the stretch in your right calf.

9 Release the stretch, and then repeat on the opposite side.

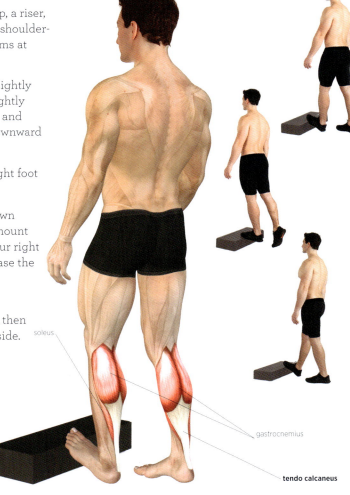

soleus

gastrocnemius

tendo calcaneus

1 MIN TARGETS

BEGINNER

3 x 10 sec holds + rest

INTERMEDIATE

3 x 15 sec holds + rest

ADVANCED

2 x 30 sec holds

BEST FOR

- Shoulders
- Hamstrings
- Back

FIND YOUR FORM

- Keep your feet flexed.
- Try sitting on a folded blanket if desired.
- To help you fold deeper onto your thighs, think of having a slight arch in your lower back as you root your thighs into the floor.

SEATED FORWARD BEND

This pose stretches your spine, shoulders, and hamstrings. It also improves digestion and stimulates internal organs such as the liver, kidneys, ovaries, and uterus. Seated Forward Bend can also ease headaches. An introspective posture, its gesture of surrender helps to reduce stress and calm your mind.

❶ Sit in Staff Pose (pages 218–19), with your legs extended in front of you and your feet flexed.

❷ Inhale and lift your arms above your head, parallel to each other. Sit up tall to lengthen your spine.

❸ Exhale and fold forward. Grasp the outside of your right foot with your right hand, and the outside of your left foot with your left hand.

❹ Hinge at your hips, easing your abdomen down toward your thighs. Allow your head to release downward, and hold for the prescribed time.

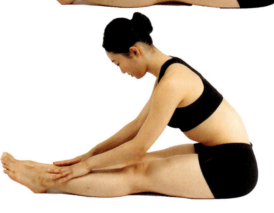

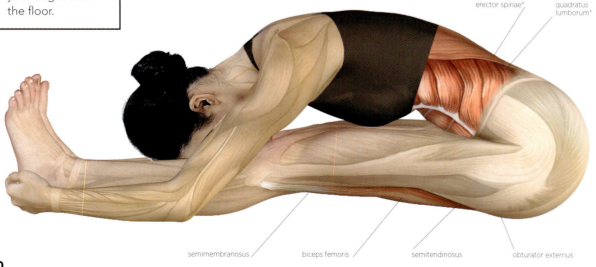

erector spinae*

quadratus lumborum*

semimembranosus   biceps femoris   semitendinosus   obturator externus

BEGINNER

4 x 10 sec holds + rest

INTERMEDIATE

4 x 15 sec holds

ADVANCED

2 x 30 sec holds

BEST FOR

- Iliotibial band
- Glutes
- Hamstrings

FIND YOUR FORM

- Keep your knees straight, yet soft, throughout the exercise.
- Let your head drop.
- Avoid bending or locking your knees.
- Avoid twisting your neck, shoulders, or torso to either side.

IT BAND STRETCH

The Garland Yoga Stretch is a popular pose in many yoga routines that provides a more intense stretch than a traditional squat. This challenging position is a deep hip opener that also lengthens your spine and strengthens your core. It improves your balance as well.

1 Stand upright, with your arms along your sides. Cross your right foot in front of your left.

2 Bending at your waist, gradually reach toward the floor with your hands.

3 Hold for the recommended time, release the stretch, and then slowly roll up to the starting position. Repeat on the opposite side.

tractus iliotibialis

vastus lateralis

semitendinosus

biceps femoris

semimembranosus

rectus femoris

gastrocnemius

soleus

1 MIN TARGETS

BEGINNER

3 x 10 secs per leg

INTERMEDIATE

2 x 15 secs per leg

ADVANCED

2 x 30 secs per leg

BEST FOR

- Quads
- Top of foot
- Ankles

FIND YOUR FORM

- Lean against a wall or other stable object with your arm opposite the bent leg to aid your balance.

- Avoid Bringing your foot closer to your buttocks than you can reach with a comfortable stretch. Unless you are extremely limber, this can compress the knee joint.

STANDING QUAD STRETCH

This stretch engages the quadriceps—the large muscle group that sits on the front of your thighs, the purpose of which is to straighten the legs and extend the knees. Be careful with this stretch if you're prone to knee or lower-back pain. If back pain is an issue for you, you can do a similar stretch while lying on your side, bending your top knee, and bringing your heel toward your buttocks. Hold onto a chair or the wall if you have trouble balancing. Doing a quad stretch after lower body exercise is key to having healthy, flexible quads.

1 Stand with your legs and feet parallel and shoulder-width apart. Bend your knees very slightly and tuck your pelvis slightly forward, lift your chest, and press your shoulders downward and back.

1 Bend your right knee behind you so that your ankle is raised toward your buttocks.

3 Bend your right knee behind you so that your ankle is raised toward your buttocks.

4 Release the stretch, switch legs, and repeat.

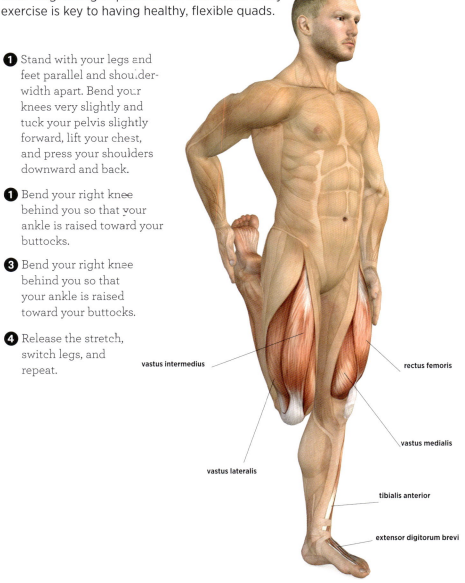

vastus intermedius

rectus femoris

vastus medialis

vastus lateralis

tibialis anterior

extensor digitorum brevi

BEGINNER

3 x 10 secs per leg

INTERMEDIATE

2 x 15 secs per leg

ADVANCED

2 x 30 secs per leg

BEST FOR

• Legs
• Core

FIND YOUR FORM

• Keep your chest up, your shoulders down, and your upper arms parallel to the floor throughout the exercise. Be sure to engage your glutes as you lunge.

• Don't crane your neck as you perform the movement. Avoid lifting your feet off the floor.

LATERAL LUNGE

The Lateral Lunge introduces a new plane of movement to lunge or squat exercises. Rather than a forward or backward motion, which takes place in the sagittal plane that divides the body into left and right, the side-to-side motion moves you in the frontal plane, which divides the body into back and front portions. A Lateral Lunge also calls for each leg to work independently, so your dominant leg cannot take on a greater share of the work. This kind of lunge has many variations that you can add to your workout regimen.

1 Stand upright with your arms outstretched in front of you, parallel to the floor.

2 Step out to the left. Squat down on your right leg, bending at your hips while maintaining a neutral spine. Begin to extend your left leg, keeping both feet flat on the floor.

3 Bend your right knee until your thigh is parallel to the floor, and your left leg is fully extended.

4 Keeping your arms parallel to the floor, squeeze your glutes and press off your right leg to return to the starting position and repeat. Perform the desired reps, then repeat on the other side.

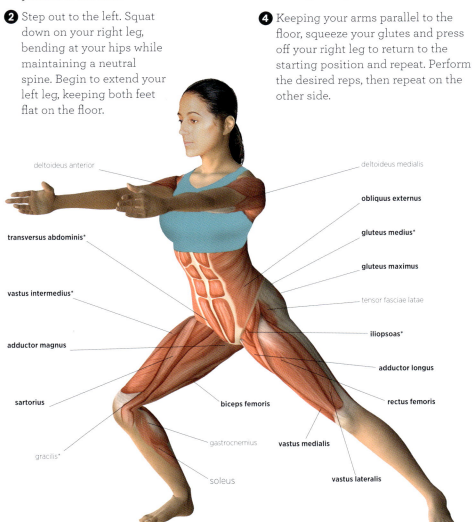

deltoideus anterior

deltoideus medialis

obliquus externus

gluteus medius*

gluteus maximus

tensor fasciae latae

transversus abdominis*

iliopsoas*

vastus intermedius*

adductor longus

adductor magnus

rectus femoris

sartorius

biceps femoris

gastrocnemius

vastus medialis

gracilis*

soleus

vastus lateralis

1 MIN TARGETS

BEGINNER
2 x 10 secs per leg

INTERMEDIATE
2 x 15 secs per leg

ADVANCED
1 x 30 secs per leg

BEST FOR

- Hamstrings
- Quadriceps
- Inner thighs
- Calves
- Obliques

FIND YOUR FORM

- Lean your back against a sofa, if necessary, to stabilize yourself and to correctly align your hip bones on the floor.
- Avoid raising your grounded thigh from the floor.

HALF STRADDLE STRETCH

The Half Straddle Stretch benefits your lower torso and your legs, opening your hips and lengthening your obliques, thighs, quads, and calves.

❶ Sit upright with your knees bent.

❷ Keeping your right knee bent, lower it to the floor, and draw your right foot in toward your groin.

❸ Extend your left leg straight out to your left side.

❹ Plant your arms on the floor behind you to support your lower back as you stretch.

❺ Hold for the recommended time, release the stretch, and then repeat on the opposite side.

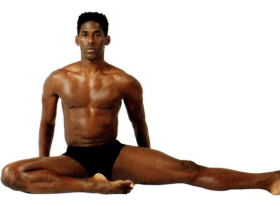

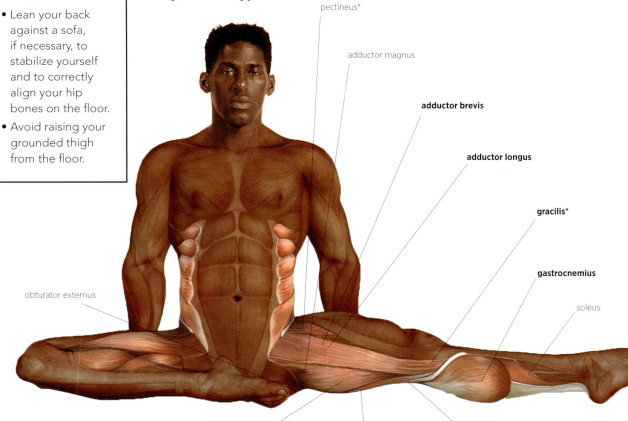

pectineus*

adductor magnus

adductor brevis

adductor longus

gracilis*

gastrocnemius

soleus

obturator externus

biceps femoris

semitendinosus

semimembranosus

BEGINNER

2 x 10 secs per leg

INTERMEDIATE

2 x 15 secs per leg

ADVANCED

1 x 30 secs per leg

BEST FOR

• Core

FIND YOUR FORM

• Engage your buttocks to maximize control over your legs.

• Keep your neck long and your shoulder blades pressed downward, away from your ears.

• Avoid Losing control of your abdominals

KNEE-TO-CHEST HUG

Knee-to-Chest Hug—the first of a group called the "stomach series"—improves your core stability while your arms and legs are moving (quickly). This exercise requires coordination, as well as control of your deep abdominal muscles. It's important to think of your powerhouse and precise positions as you perform this exercise, so that your legs and torso don't begin to tip and tilt like a rowboat in a storm at sea.

1 Lie on your back with your legs in tabletop position, your spine extended along the floor and your knees bent so that your legs form a 90-degree angle, feet flexed. Your neck should be long, your throat open, your shoulder blades stabilized, and your arms extended along your sides, palms down.

2 To prepare, inhale while curling the top of your head forward so that you are looking between your knees. Place your hands on the outsides of your calves.

3 Exhale, and extend one leg diagonally to form a 45-degree angle with the floor, bringing your outside hand to your ankle and your inside hand to your knee.

4 Inhale, and begin to switch hands and legs.

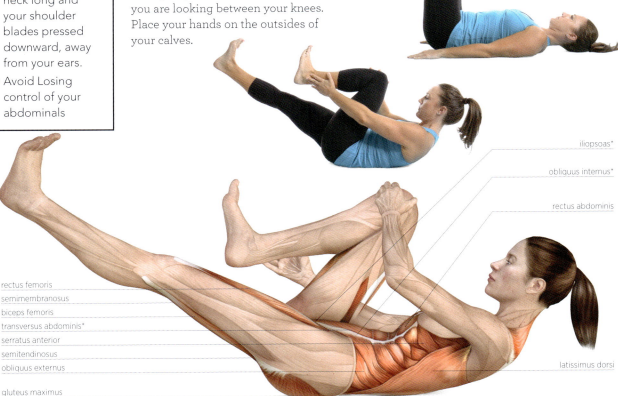

iliopsoas*

obliquus internus*

rectus abdominis

rectus femoris

semimembranosus

biceps femoris

transversus abdominis*

serratus anterior

semitendinosus

obliquus externus

gluteus maximus

latissimus dorsi

1 MIN TARGETS

BEGINNER

Repeat for 1 min

INTERMEDIATE

Repeat for 90 secs

ADVANCED

Repeat for 2+ mins

BEST FOR

• Neck
• Shoulders
• Scapulae

FIND YOUR FORM

• Move in a smooth, controlled manner.
• Avoid rolling your shoulders.

SHRUG

It might seem like we shrug all the time, but purposefully engaging the shrug muscles can be an effective means to strengthen the neck, upper back, and shoulders.

1 Sit on a Swiss ball or chair. Keep your back straight and your head and neck centered over the rest of your spinal column.

2 With your arms at your sides, bend your elbows slightly. Hold your hands with the palms up.

3 Bring your shoulders down and forward, and then lift them as high as you can.

4 Return the starting position, and then repeat for the recommended repetitions.

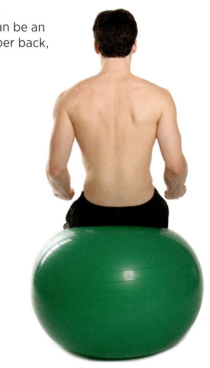

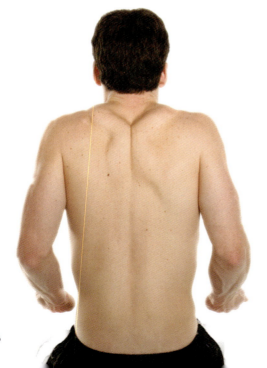

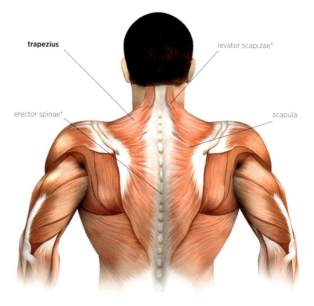

trapezius

levator scapulae*

erector spinae*

scapula

BEGINNER

4 x 10 sec holds + rest

INTERMEDIATE

4 x 15 sec holds

ADVANCED

2 x 30 sec holds

BEST FOR

- Spine
- Shoulders
- Glutes

FIND YOUR FORM

- Apply gentle pressure between your elbows and your knees, encouraging your knees to open farther and deepening the inner-thigh stretch.
- Lengthen your spine, keeping your back straight.
- Broaden across your collarbones.
- Avoid rounding your shoulders forward.

COBRA STRETCH

As well as promoting spinal flexibility, this yoga-inspired stretch builds strength in your back and shoulders and also in your abdominals, buttocks, and chest.

1 Lie facedown. Bend your elbows, placing your hands flat on the floor beside your chest. Extend your legs, and press down into the floor with your thighs and the tops of your feet.

2 Inhaling, lift your chest off the floor, pressing your palms downward.

3 Continue lifting your chest as you straighten your arms.

4 Hold for the recommended time, and then, on an exhalation, lower yourself to the floor.

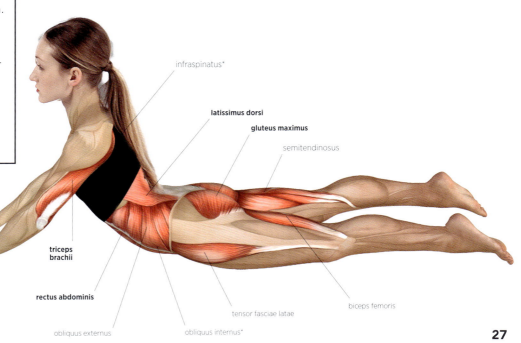

infraspinatus*

latissimus dorsi

gluteus maximus

semitendinosus

triceps brachii

rectus abdominis

biceps femoris

tensor fasciae latae

obliquus externus

obliquus internus*

1 MIN TARGETS

BEGINNER
5 x 5 secs per side

INTERMEDIATE
4 x 10 secs per side

ADVANCED
2 x 30 secs oer side

BEST FOR

- Shoulders
- Chest
- Legs
- Spine

FIND YOUR FORM

- Keep your leading knee tight and aligned with the center of your foot, shin, and thigh.
- If you feel unsteady, brace your back heel against a wall.
- Avoid twisting your hips.

TRIANGLE YOGA STRETCH

A classic yoga pose, the Triangle stretches your torso and spine while mobilizing your hips. It also strengthens your core and helps you focus on the correct alignment of your shoulders.

1 Stand with your feet slightly farther than shoulder-width apart.

2 Inhale, and raise both arms straight out to your sides, keeping them parallel to the floor. Your palms should be facing down.

3 Exhale slowly, and without bending your knees, pivot on your heels and turn your right foot to your right and your left foot slightly toward your right, keeping your heels in line with each other.

4 Lean your torso to your right side as far as is comfortable, keeping your arms parallel to the floor.

5 Drop your right arm and rest your right hand on your shin or ankle.
At the same time, extend your left arm straight up toward the ceiling.

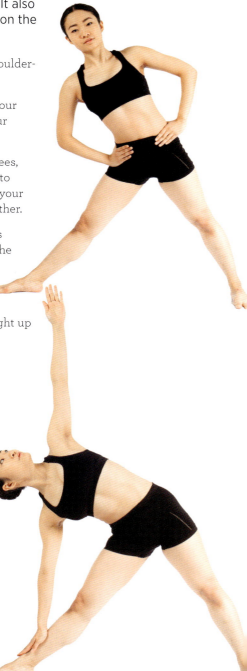

6 Gently twist your spine and torso counterclockwise, using your extended arms as levers, while your spinal axis remains parallel to the floor. Pull your arms away from each other in opposite directions. Turn your head to gaze at your left thumb, slightly intensifying the twist in your spine.

7 Hold for the recommended time. Inhale, as you return to the standing position with your arms outstretched, strongly pressing your back heel into the floor. Reverse your foot position, and then repeat on the opposite side.

MODIFICATION

HARDER: Stretch your legs farther apart, von the floor next to the outside of your extended foot.

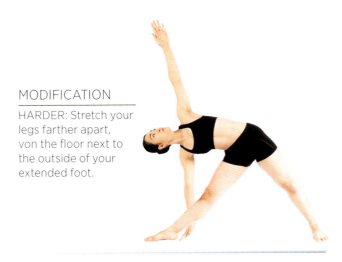

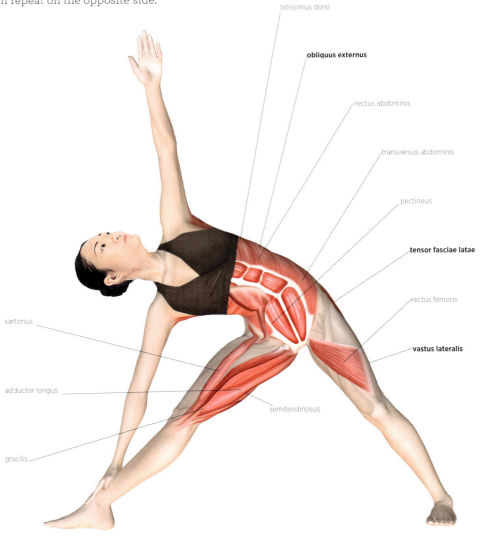

latissimus dorsi

obliquus externus

rectus abdominis

transversus abdominis

pectineus

tensor fasciae latae

rectus femoris

vastus lateralis

sartorius

adductor longus

semitendinosus

gracilis

1 MIN TARGETS

BEGINNER
3 x 10 secs per side

INTERMEDIATE
2 x 15 secs per side

ADVANCED
2 x 30 secs per side

BEST FOR

- Abdominals
- Shoulders
- Obliques

FIND YOUR FORM

- Squat deep, and be sure to keep your thighs parallel to the floor.
- Avoid hyperextending your knees past your toes while squatting.

DIAGONAL REACH

The Diagonal Reach strengthens your abdominal muscles and stretches your obliques along the sides of your body. It also works your shoulders and arms. Move smoothly and fully extend your arms to deepen the stretch.

1 Stand with your feet hip-width apart and your arms at your sides.

2 Raise your arms diagonally upward and to your right. Follow your hands with your gaze.

3 Hold for the recommended time, release the stretch, and then repeat on the opposite side. Perform the recommended repetitions.

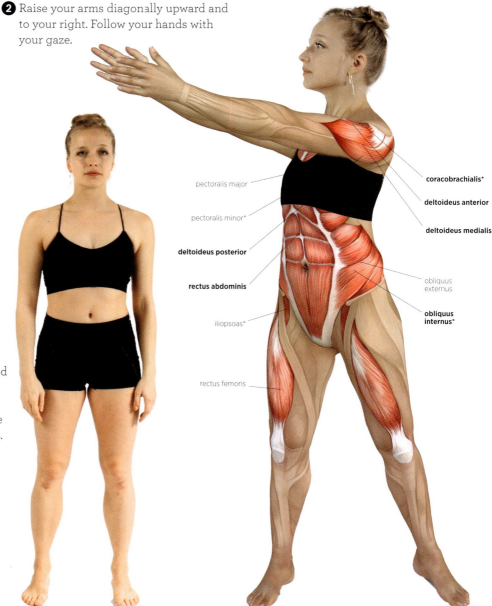

pectoralis major

pectoralis minor*

deltoideus posterior

rectus abdominis

iliopsoas*

rectus femoris

coracobrachialis*

deltoideus anterior

deltoideus medialis

obliquus externus

obliquus internus*

BEGINNER

3 x 10 secs per side

INTERMEDIATE

2 x 15 secs per side

ADVANCED

2 x 30 secs per side

BEST FOR

• Neck
• Shoulders

FIND YOUR FORM

• Apply only a gentle pressure.
• Avoid any movement in the neck.

LATERAL ISOMETRIC STRETCH

This stretch helps you maintain or regain cervical mobility simply by applying pressure while you move your neck through its normal movements. Perform this stretch slowly and gently to ease and release the top of your shoulders and lower-neck muscles.

❶ Sit or stand, keeping your neck, shoulders, and torso straight. Place the palm of your right hand on the top of your head.

❷ Reach toward the small of your back with your left hand, bending your arm at the elbow.

❸ Tilt your head toward your raised elbow until you feel the stretch in the side of your neck.

❹ Press your head into the palm of your hand as you try to tilt your ear to your shoulder.

❺ Hold for the recommended time, release the stretch, and then repeat on the opposite side. Alternate sides for the recommended repetitions.

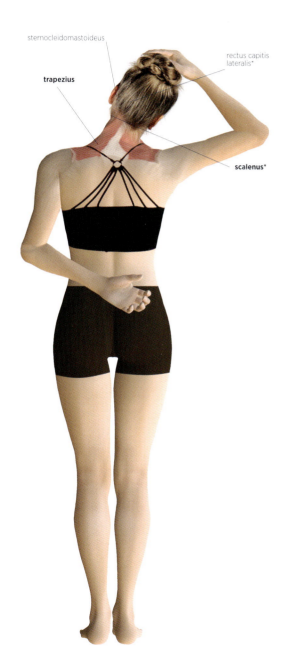

sternocleidomastoideus

rectus capitis lateralis*

trapezius

scalenus*

1 MIN TARGETS

BEGINNER

3 x 10 sec holds + rest

INTERMEDIATE

3 x 15 sec holds + rest

ADVANCED

2 x 30 sec holds

BEST FOR

• Abdominals

FIND YOUR FORM

• Position your legs on the ball to form a 45-degree angle with the rest of your body before you curl.

• Move smoothly, maintaining control of the ball.

• Keep your arms anchored to the floor.

• Engage your abdominals, and squeeze your glutes.

• Avoid arching your back in the curl position.

SWISS BALL HAMSTRINGS CURL

The Swiss Ball Hamstrings Curl is a challenging exercise that targets your hamstrings and glutes. Choose a ball size that you are comfortable with, keeping in mind that the larger the ball the greater the muscle contraction.

1 Lie on your back with your arms along your sides, angled slightly away from your body. Extend your legs, and rest your lower legs and ankles on top of a Swiss ball.

2 Pressing downward with your feet, bend your knees as you roll the ball toward you. Curl your pelvis, and raise your lower body off the floor. Hold for a few moments.

3 With control, return to the starting position. Repeat for the recommended repetitions.

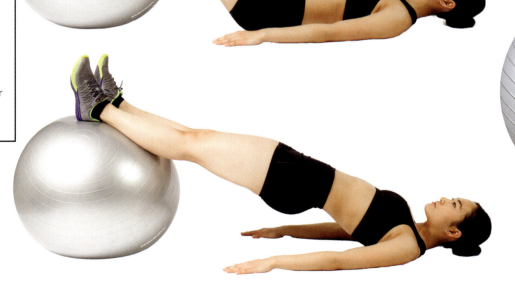

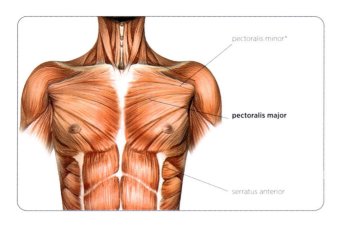

pectoralis minor*

pectoralis major

serratus anterior

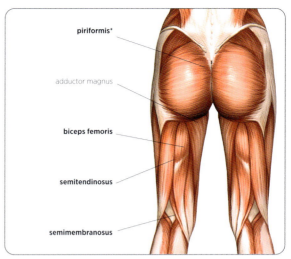

piriformis*

adductor magnus

biceps femoris

semitendinosus

semimembranosus

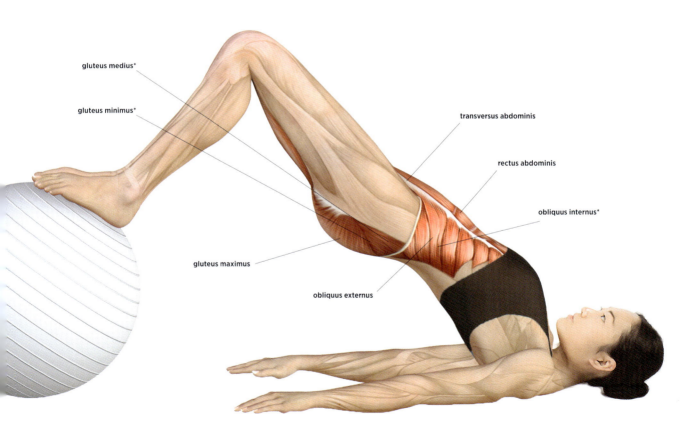

gluteus medius*

gluteus minimus*

gluteus maximus

obliquus externus

transversus abdominis

rectus abdominis

obliquus internus*

1 MIN TARGETS

BEGINNER

3 x 10 secs per side

INTERMEDIATE

2 x 15 secs per side

ADVANCED

2 x 30 secs per side

BEST FOR

- Chest
- Upper back
- Obliques

FIND YOUR FORM

- Keep your hips planted firmly on the floor.
- Use your legs to anchor your body.
- Lengthen your neck.
- Avoid hunching your shoulders.
- Avoid rolling your hips.

SAW STRETCH

This classic Pilates exercise uses oppositional movement to stretch your chest and upper back. The Saw improves flexibility in the spine and strengthens your abdominal obliques. This exercise helps you focus on stabilizing your pelvis during rotation.

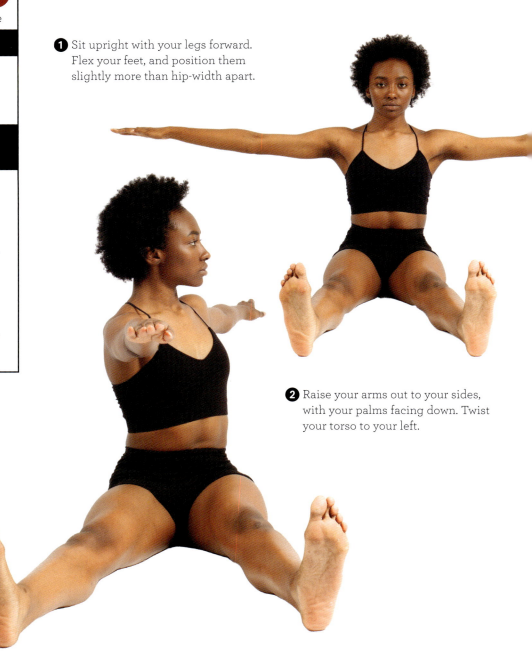

❶ Sit upright with your legs forward. Flex your feet, and position them slightly more than hip-width apart.

❷ Raise your arms out to your sides, with your palms facing down. Twist your torso to your left.

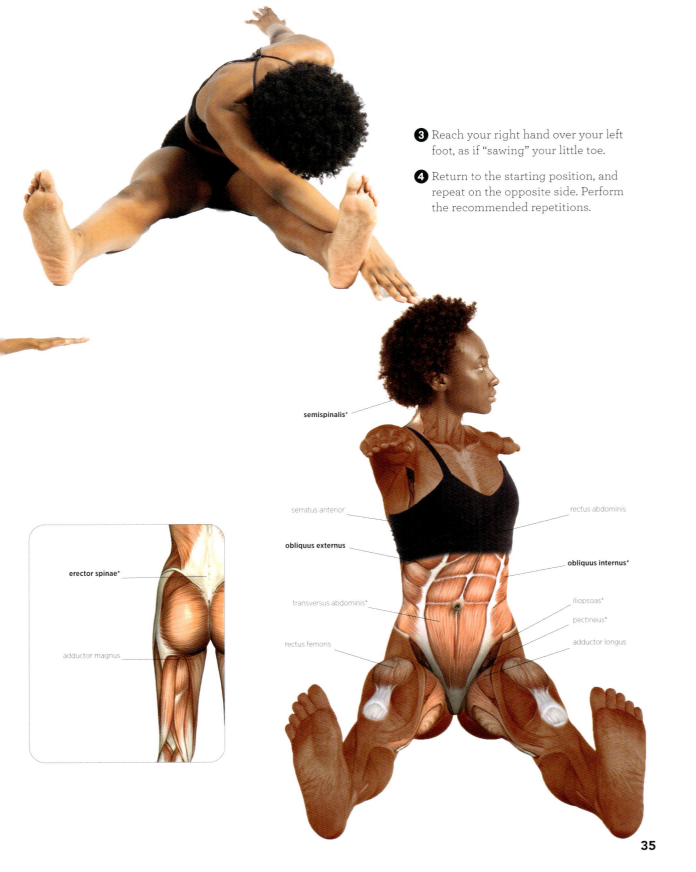

3 Reach your right hand over your left foot, as if "sawing" your little toe.

4 Return to the starting position, and repeat on the opposite side. Perform the recommended repetitions.

semispinalis*

serratus anterior

obliquus externus

transversus abdominis*

rectus femoris

rectus abdominis

obliquus internus*

iliopsoas*

pectineus*

adductor longus

erector spinae*

adductor magnus

1 MIN TARGETS

BEGINNER

4 x 10 sec holds + rest

INTERMEDIATE

3 x 15 sec holds

ADVANCED

3 x 30 sec holds

BEST FOR

- Abs
- Back
- Thighs

FIND YOUR FORM

- Keep your abdominals flat throughout the exercise.
- Extend your legs only to an angle at which you can maintain torso stability.
- Keep your chin slightly tilted toward your chest.
- Avoid arching your back.
- Avoid rolling your shoulders forward.
- Avoid straining your neck.

DOUBLE-LEG STRETCH

Double-Leg Stretch is the first of the classical Pilates stomach series. It works your powerhouse muscles, stretches your body, and develops coordination. Once you feel comfortable doing it along with Single-Leg Stretch, you will be able to easily flow between them. The closer your extended arms and legs are to the floor, the harder it is to stabilize your torso—so start by lowering only to the level that you can control comfortably.

1 Lie on your back in tabletop position, with your spine extended along the floor and your bent legs forming a 90-degree angle. Make sure your neck is long and your throat open. Your shoulder blades should be stabilized down your back. Extend your arms along your sides.

2 Inhale as you begin to peel your upper body off the floor and forward toward your knees. Place your hands on the outsides of your calves.

3 Engage your lower abdominals, exhale, and lengthen your torso, extending your arms overhead to a position parallel to your ears. At the same time, extend your legs to a 45-degree angle above your mat.

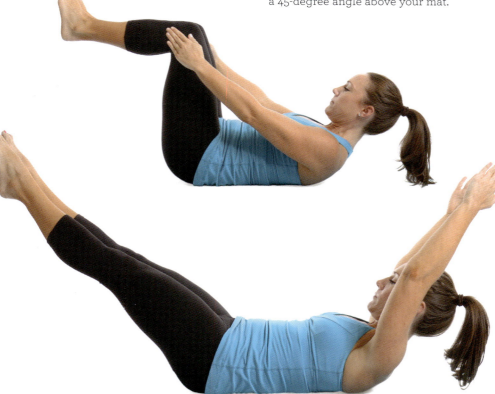

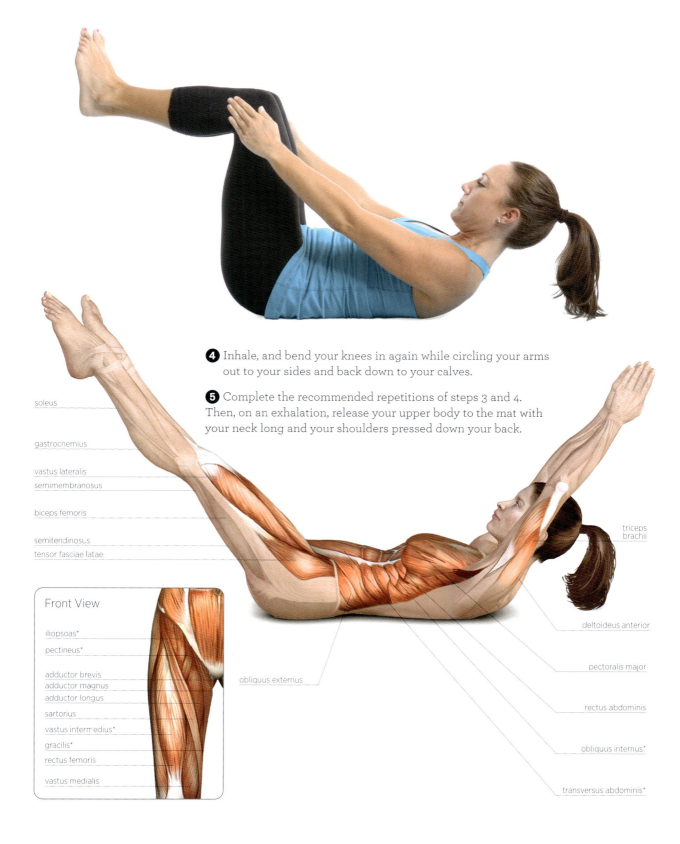

4 Inhale, and bend your knees in again while circling your arms out to your sides and back down to your calves.

5 Complete the recommended repetitions of steps 3 and 4. Then, on an exhalation, release your upper body to the mat with your neck long and your shoulders pressed down your back.

soleus

gastrocnemius

vastus lateralis
semimembranosus

biceps femoris

semitendinosus
tensor fasciae latae

triceps
brachii

deltoideus anterior

pectoralis major

rectus abdominis

obliquus internus*

obliquus externus

transversus abdominis*

Front View

iliopsoas*

pectineus*

adductor brevis
adductor magnus
adductor longus
sartorius
vastus intermedius*
gracilis*
rectus femoris
vastus medialis

1 MIN TARGETS

BEGINNER
3 x 10 secs per side

INTERMEDIATE
2 x 15 secs per side

ADVANCED
2 x 30 secs per side

BEST FOR

• Triceps
• Shoulders

FIND YOUR FORM

• Keep your shoulders pressed down and back, away from your ears.

• Maintain a firm, stable midsection, keeping your pelvis slightly tucked.

• Avoid tilting your head or neck forward.

TRICEPS STRETCH

The Triceps Stretch is easy to do anytime, anywhere. It improves shoulder and upper-body flexibility, fends off muscle soreness, and extends your range of motion while building durability.

1 Stand with your legs and feet parallel and shoulder-width apart. Bend your knees very slightly, and shift your pelvis slightly forward.

2 Reach your right arm up behind your head. Bend from the elbow, aiming to bring your elbow toward the middle of the back of your head. Your right hand should fall between your shoulder blades

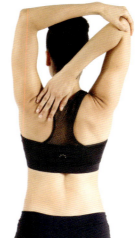 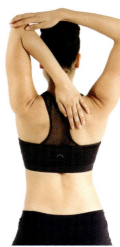

3 Grab your right elbow with your left hand, and gently pull down to intensify the stretch.

4 Hold for the recommended time, release the stretch, and then repeat on the opposite side.

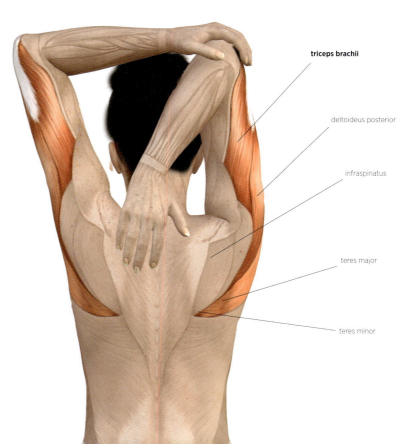

triceps brachii

deltoideus posterior

infraspinatus

teres major

teres minor

BEGINNER

4 x 10 sec holds + rest

INTERMEDIATE

3 x 15 sec holds

ADVANCED

3 x 30 sec holds

BEST FOR

- Shoulders
- Chest

FIND YOUR FORM

- Keep your shoulders pressed down and back, away from your ears.
- Avoid collapsing your chest forward.

BICEPS AND PECS STRETCH

This stretch opens up the upper-front part of your body. Working the chest and upper arms together, it counteracts tightening caused by bad habits such as slouching.

1 Stand with your legs and feet parallel and shoulder-width apart. Shift your pelvis slightly forward.

2 Clasp your hands together behind your back with your fingers interwoven. If you want an extra stretch, twist your hands and wrists so that your palms are pulled in toward your buttocks and your thumbs point downward.

3 Hold for the recommended time, release the stretch, and then repeat for the recommended repetitions.

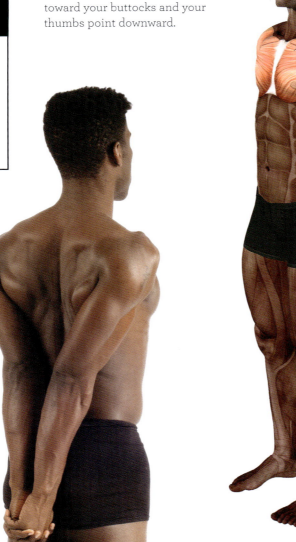

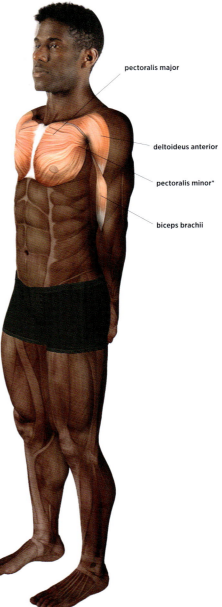

pectoralis major

deltoideus anterior

pectoralis minor*

biceps brachii

1 MIN TARGETS

BEGINNER

3 x 10 secs per side

INTERMEDIATE

2 x 15 secs per side

ADVANCED

2 x 30 secs per side

BEST FOR

• Chest
• Shoulders

FIND YOUR FORM

• Keep your shoulders pressed down and back, away from your ears.

• Position the arm against the wall so that your elbow is slightly lower than your shoulder and your wrist is slightly below your elbow, at a slight diagonal, to protect your rotator cuff from injury.

• Avoid rotating your chest and/or torso toward the wall when lunging; instead, face forward.

WALL-ASSISTED CHEST STRETCH

To really target each side of your body, you can't go wrong with the wall-assisted chest stretch.

❶ Stand parallel to a wall, with the wall on the left side of your body.

❷ Extend your left arm back against the wall, so that your palm is flat against it.

❸ Lunge forward with your left foot.

❹ Remain facing forward as you stretch. To stay aware of any torso twisting, place your right hand just below your left pectoral muscle, fingers on your rib cage

❺ Return to the starting position, turn so that the wall is on your right, and repeat.

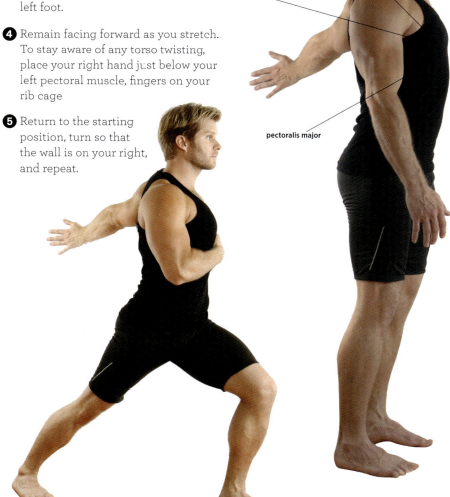

pectoralis minor*

deltoideus anterior

pectoralis major

BEGINNER

2 x 10 secs per leg

INTERMEDIATE

2 x 15 secs per leg

ADVANCED

1 x 30 secs per leg

BEST FOR

• piriformis
• glutes
• lower back

FIND YOUR FORM

• Be sure to ease into the movement slowly.

• Relax your hips to enable a deeper stretch.

• Avoid pulling your thigh to your chest forcefully or jerkily.

PIRIFORMIS STRETCH

This move targets the gluteal and hip regions, and takes around two minutes to complete. The piriformis muscle laterally rotates and stabilizes the hip, and is particularly used in sports that require sudden changes of direction.

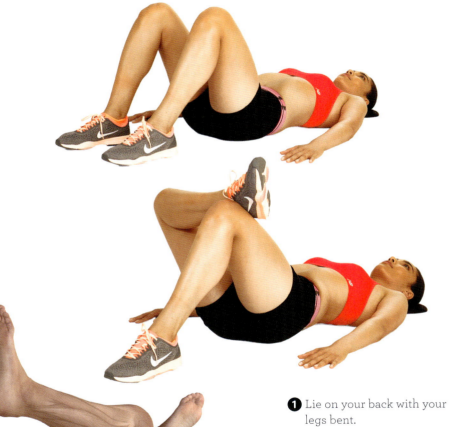

piriformis*

gluteus minimus*

gluteus maximus

quadratus femoris*

❶ Lie on your back with your legs bent.

❷ Cross your right ankle over your left knee.

❸ Use your hands to grab the back of the left thigh close to the knee, and gently pull it toward your right shoulder. Hold for 30 seconds, relax, and then hold for another 30 seconds, then switch sides.

41

LEGS

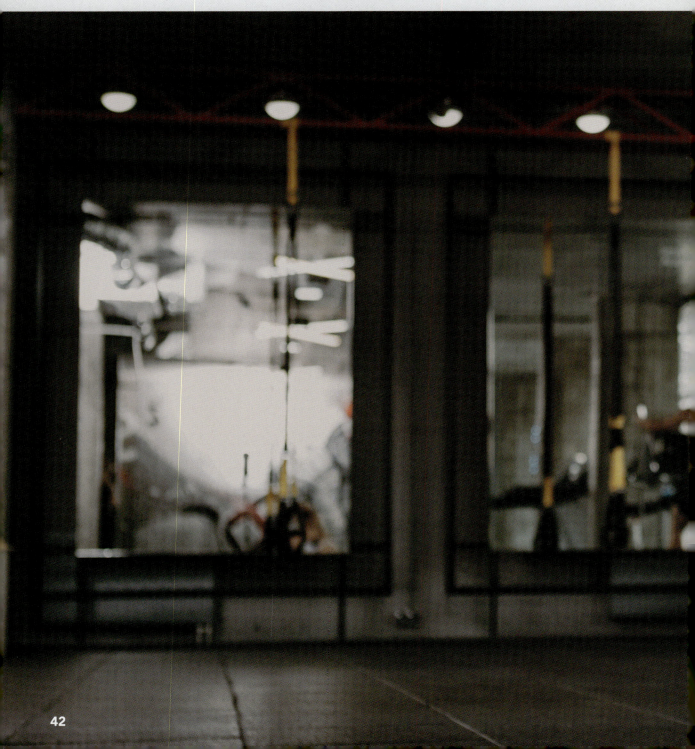

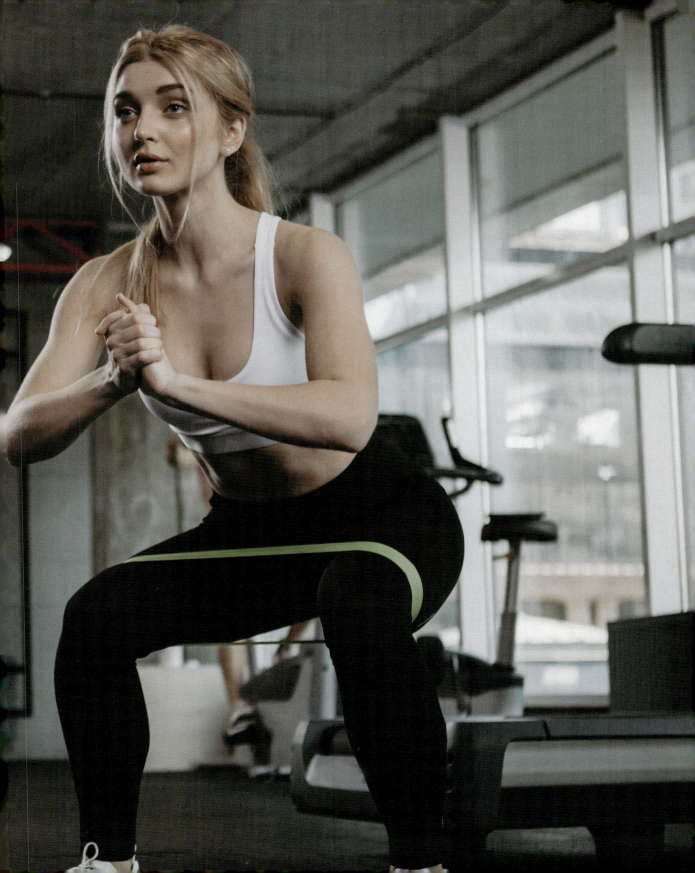

1 MIN TARGETS

BEGINNER

4 x 10 sec holds + rest

INTERMEDIATE

4 x 15 sec holds

ADVANCED

3 x 30 sec holds

BEST FOR

- Hips
- Lower legs
- Quads

FIND YOUR FORM

- Imagine pressing into the floor as you rise from the squat, creating your body's own resistance in your leg muscles.

SQUAT

The Squat integrates balance, coordination, resistance, and stretching to target your leg muscles. This exercise also strengthens the muscles of your feet.

1 Stand with your legs and feet parallel and shoulder-width apart, and your knees bent very slightly. Tuck your pelvis slightly forward, lift your chest, and press your shoulders downward and back.

2 Extend your arms in front of your body for stability, keeping them even with your shoulders. Plant your feet firmly on the floor, and curl your toes slightly upward.

3 Draw in your abdominal muscles and bend into a squat. Keep your heels planted on the floor and your chest as upright as possible, resisting the urge to bend too far forward.

4 Exhale, and return to the original position. Repeat five to six times.

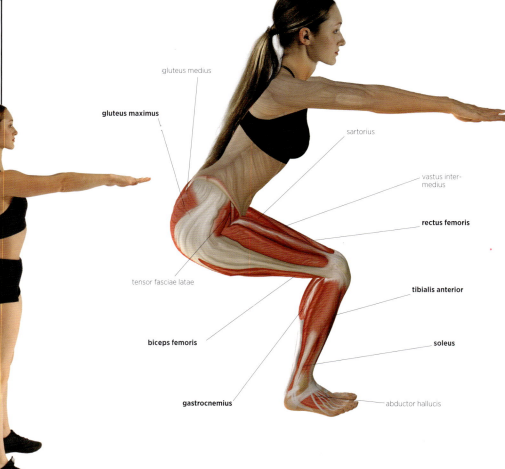

gluteus medius

gluteus maximus

sartorius

vastus inter-medius

rectus femoris

tensor fasciae latae

tibialis anterior

biceps femoris

soleus

gastrocnemius

abductor hallucis

BEGINNER

4 x 10 sec holds + rest

INTERMEDIATE

4 x 15 sec holds

ADVANCED

3 x 30 sec holds

BEST FOR

• Inner thighs

FIND YOUR FORM

• Imagine that you are balancing a book on top of your head. This will help you keep your chest elevated and the weight of your upper body over your hips.

• Avoid leaning your torso forward.

SUMO SQUAT

Like any squat, the Sumo Squat is a terrific lower-body exercise that tones your thighs, butt, and calves. Its execution is similar to a Basic Squat, but your stance is wider and your toes are sharply angled away from the midline of your body. This kind of squat—which gets its name from the stance of a Japanese sumo wrestler— adds an inner-thigh focus to your workout. There are many variations, including weighted ones.

1 Stand with your feet planted beyond shoulder width and your toes turned out. Bend your knees very slightly and tuck your pelvis slightly forward, lift your chest, and press your shoulders downward and back.

2 Place your hands on your thighs.

3 Squat down until your thighs are parallel to the floor, keeping your weight on your heels.

4 Push off with your heels at the bottom of the squat, squeezing your glutes and inner thighs to rise back to the starting position.

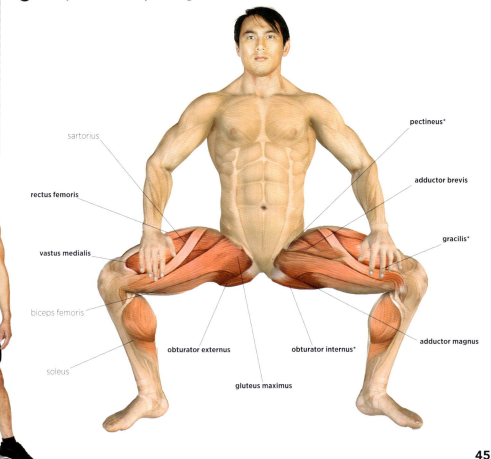

sartorius

rectus femoris

vastus medialis

biceps femoris

soleus

obturator externus

gluteus maximus

obturator internus*

pectineus*

adductor brevis

gracilis*

adductor magnus

1 MIN TARGETS

BEGINNER
4 x 10 sec holds + rest

INTERMEDIATE
4 x 15 sec holds

ADVANCED
3 x 30 sec holds

BEST FOR

- Calves
- Glutes
- Quadriceps
- Hamstrings
- Shoulders
- Upper back

FIND YOUR FORM

- Keep your back straight and your core upright.
- Press your shoulders back and down.
- Avoid arching your back as you raise your arms.
- Avoid letting your abdominals bulge outward.

SPLIT SQUAT WITH OVERHEAD PRESS

A multipurpose exercise, the Split Squat with Overhead Press combines the single-leg strengthening move of a staggered-stance squat with the upper-body toning of an upward press. This exercise will challenge your quads, glutes, hamstrings, upper back, and shoulders.

1 Stand with your right leg behind you with the ball of your foot resting on a step.

2 With your elbows bent to form right angles, raise both arms to shoulder height. Position your hands as if your were grasping a bar using an overhand grip.

3 Bend both knees into a split squat position. Simultaneously, extend your arms over your head.

4 Return to the starting position, and then repeat on the opposite side. Repeat for the recommended repetitions.

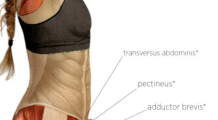

triceps brachii
anterior deltoid
posterior deltoid
medial deltoid
transversus abdominis*
pectineus*
adductor brevis*
rectus femoris
vastus medialis
tensor fasciae latae
gastrocnemius
gracilis*
vastus intermedius*
soleus
vastus lateralis

BEGINNER

3 x 10 secs per leg

INTERMEDIATE

2 x 15 secs per leg

ADVANCED

2 x 30 secs per leg

BEST FOR

• Thighs
• Calves
• Glutes

FIND YOUR FORM

• Bring your abdomen in, away from your thigh.

• Keep your hips firm as you stretch.

• Roll the inner thigh of your straight leg toward the ceiling, finding its internal rotation.

• Place your hands on blocks to help elongate your spine if your back begins rounding when your fingertips touch the floor.

• Avoid positioning your knee past your ankle and over your toes, which can stress your knee joint.

LUNGE

An integral component of many yoga flows, Lunge provides a smooth transition to or from forward bends or arm supports, such as Downward-Facing Dog. Like other lunges, it strengthens the lower body, especially the thighs.

1 Begin in Downward-Facing Dog. Step your left foot forward in between your hands, with your left knee and shin lined up over your left ankle.

2 With your fingertips resting on the floor, square your hips to the front of the mat, grounding your left heel into the floor and drawing your left hip crease back.

3 Extend your right leg straight behind you, resting the ball of your foot on the mat. Lengthen all the way from the crown of your head to your right heel. Gaze slightly ahead, keeping the back of your neck long.

4 Hold as recommended, and then repeat on the other side.

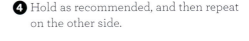

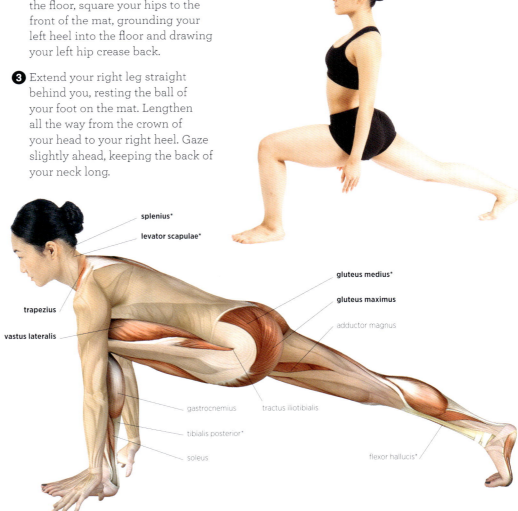

splenius*

levator scapulae*

gluteus medius*

gluteus maximus

adductor magnus

trapezius

vastus lateralis

gastrocnemius

tractus iliotibialis

tibialis posterior*

soleus

flexor hallucis*

1 MIN TARGETS

BEGINNER
3 x 10 secs per leg

INTERMEDIATE
2 x 15 secs per leg

ADVANCED
2 x 30 secs per leg

BEST FOR

• Thighs
• Glutes
• Calves

FIND YOUR FORM

• Tuck in your belly, away from your thigh.
• Keep your hips firm as you stretch.
• Roll the inner thigh of your straight leg toward the ceiling, finding its internal rotation.
• Place your hands on blocks to help elongate your spine if your back begins rounding when your fingertips touch the floor.
• Avoid positioning your knee past your ankle and over your toes, which can stress your knee joint.

DEEP LUNGE

This version of a forward lunge is often called High Lunge in yoga, and is also known as a Low Forward Lunge. It is an effective leg and arm strengthener that targets your glutes and quadriceps, along with your hamstrings and calf muscles. The deep position also lengthens your groin muscles.

1 Begin in Downward-Facing Dog. Step your right foot forward in between your hands, with your right knee and shin in lined with your right ankle.

2 With your fingertips resting on the floor, square your hips, grounding your right heel into the floor and drawing your right hip crease back.

3 Extend your left leg straight behind you, resting the ball of your foot on the floor. Lengthen all the way from the crown of your head to your left heel. Gaze slightly ahead, keeping the back of your neck long.

4 Hold as recommended, then repeat on the opposite side.

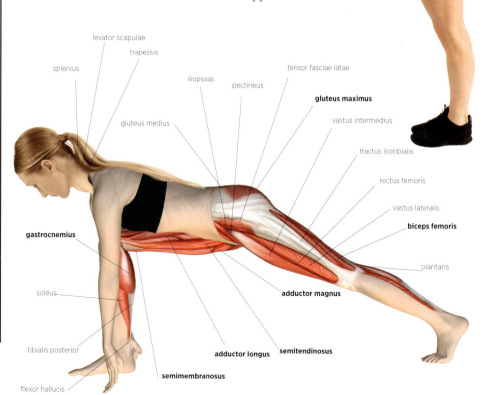

levator scapulae
trapezius
splenius
iliopsoas
pectineus
tensor fasciae latae
gluteus maximus
gluteus medius
vastus intermedius
tractus iliotibialis
rectus femoris
vastus lateralis
biceps femoris
plantaris
gastrocnemius
adductor magnus
soleus
semitendinosus
tibialis posterior
adductor longus
semimembranosus
flexor hallucis

Like the Forward Lunge, the Walking Lunge is a dynamic stretch that stabilizes your knees while building strength in your thigh muscles, both front and back. The Walking Lunge also efficiently works your glutes to firm and lift your butt, and the forward progression adds cardio intensity.

1 Stand with your legs together and your arms hanging at your sides.

2 Take a large step forward with your left leg.

3 Lower your right knee to the floor, and then forcefully push off your left foot to return to standing position. Repeat on the other side, and continue to alternate your leading leg as you move forward for the desired steps.

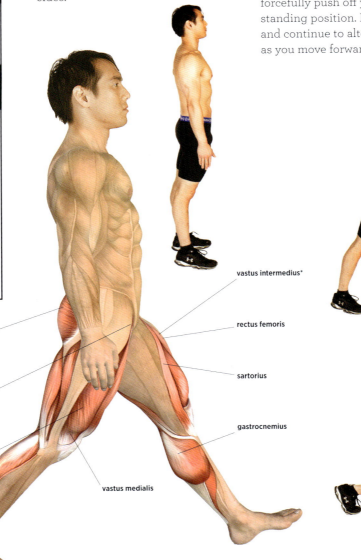

vastus intermedius*

rectus femoris

sartorius

gastrocnemius

gluteus maximus

iliopsoas*

vastus lateralis

vastus medialis

1 MIN TARGETS

BEGINNER
3 x 10 secs per leg

INTERMEDIATE
2 x 15 secs per leg

ADVANCED
2 x 30 secs per leg

BEST FOR

- Thighs
- Core
- Calves

FIND YOUR FORM

- To fully engage your glutes, press the heel of your front foot into the floor as you lift up.
- Avoid extending your front knee past your toes.

REVERSE LUNGE

Like the Forward Lunge, the Reverse Lunge is an excellent lower-body exercise. Also known as the Step-Back Lunge, this lunge variation offers your body a challenge by moving you backward—a direction you probably don't move in very often. Some proponents prefer this version over its opposite, because its backward momentum keeps your body in the optimal lunge position—your weight is on your heel with your knee above your ankle. This is a great exercise to prepare you for sports and other activities that require speed and power, particularly sprinting, but it is also the less difficult of the two basic lunges, and it is often a good option for anyone with a balance problem.

1 Stand with your hands on your hips and your feet shoulder-width apart.

2 Take a big step backward, bending your knees as you do so.

3 When your front thigh is roughly parallel to the floor, push through your front heel to return to the starting position.

4 Switch legs, and repeat on the other side.

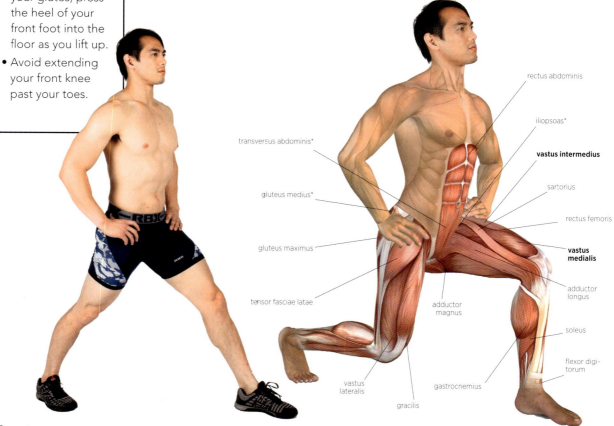

rectus abdominis

iliopsoas*

vastus intermedius

transversus abdominis*

sartorius

gluteus medius*

rectus femoris

gluteus maximus

vastus medialis

adductor longus

tensor fasciae latae

adductor magnus

soleus

flexor digitorum

vastus lateralis

gastrocnemius

gracilis

BEGINNER

3 x 10 sec holds + rest

INTERMEDIATE

3 x 15 sec holds + rest

ADVANCED

2 x 30 sec holds

BEST FOR

- Abdominals
- Glutes
- Back
- Hamstrings

FIND YOUR FORM

- While holding Dolphin Pose, keep your back straight. If you cannot straighten your legs without sagging or rounding your spine, keep your knees slightly bent.
- Avoid raising your heels off the mat.

DOLPHIN PIKE

Dolphin Pike is known to strengthen both your upper and lower body—your shoulders, arms, abdominals, and spine, as well as your thighs and calves. This energizing posture also helps you improve your balance.

1 Kneel on the floor with your hips lifted off your heels.

2 Bend forward and place your hands on the mat in front of you; lower your elbows to the floor, keeping them tucked in at your sides and aligned with your shoulders.

3 Straighten your legs as you lift your sit bones toward the ceiling. Tuck your tailbone toward your pubis, and squeeze your legs together.

4 Push through your forearms, and extend the stretch through your shoulders. Keep your head and chest lifted off the mat.

5 Hold and repeat as recommended.

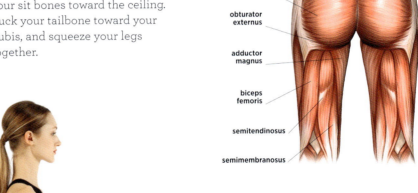

gluteus maximus
obturator externus
adductor magnus
biceps femoris
semitendinosus
semimembranosus

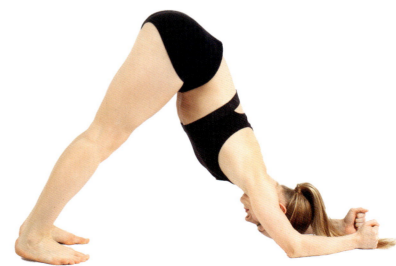

1 MIN TARGETS

BEGINNER

3 x 10 secs per leg

INTERMEDIATE

2 x 15 secs per leg

ADVANCED

2 x 30 secs per leg

BEST FOR

- Glutes
- Thighs
- Back
- Shoulders

FIND YOUR FORM

- Keep your shoulders pressed downward.
- Keep your neck relaxed.
- Keep your upper body upright as you rise up and lower yourself down.
- Avoid twisting either hip.
- Avoid hunching your shoulders.
- Avoid arching your back or hunching forward.

LATERAL EXTENSION REVERSE LUNGE

Backward lunges can be easier than forward ones because your knees take less strain, plus keeping your weight on your forward leg stabilizes the pose. This exercise is certainly great for the glutes, quads, and hamstrings.

1 Stand with your feet a little way apart, up to hip-width, and your arms at the sides of your body or with your hands on your hips.

2 Step your right leg backward. Keep a slight bend in your right knee and rest the ball of your foot on the floor.

3 Bend both knees as you move into a lunge position. Lower your body, flexing your left knee and hip until your right leg is almost in contact with the floor. Raise your arms to the sides until they are level with your shoulders.

4 Return to the starting position by straightening out your left leg and bringing your right leg forward to meet your left.

5 Switch legs and repeat on the opposite side. Alternate sides for the recommended repetitions.

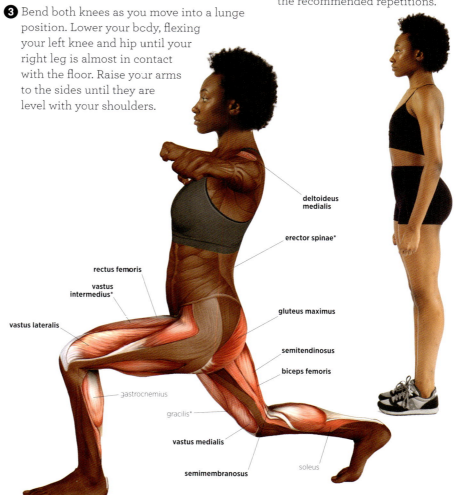

deltoideus medialis

erector spinae*

rectus femoris

vastus intermedius*

vastus lateralis

gluteus maximus

semitendinosus

biceps femoris

gastrocnemius

gracilis*

vastus medialis

soleus

semimembranosus

BEGINNER

6 x 5 secs per leg

INTERMEDIATE

10 x 5 secs per leg

ADVANCED

20 x 5 secs per leg

BEST FOR

• Thighs
• IT Bands
• Hips

FIND YOUR FORM

• Push through your heels to drive the exercise, moving with control and keeping a steady, quick pace.
• Avoid hyperextending your knee past your toes.

SKATER'S LUNGE

The high-energy Skater targets your inner and outer thighs, including your hip adductor and abductor muscles and iliotibial bands, which all work to keep your knees and hips stable. Try it if you are a runner: it counterbalances the effects of repetitive flexion and extension, alleviating the resulting strength imbalance between the inner- and outer-thigh muscles and the quadriceps and hamstrings.

❶ Stand with your legs spaced wider than shoulder-width apart and your toes pointing forward.

❷ Slide to your side into a side lunge as you bend forward slightly with your hands placed on your thigh, and then move in the opposite direction.

❸ Slide back and forth for the desired time or repetitions.

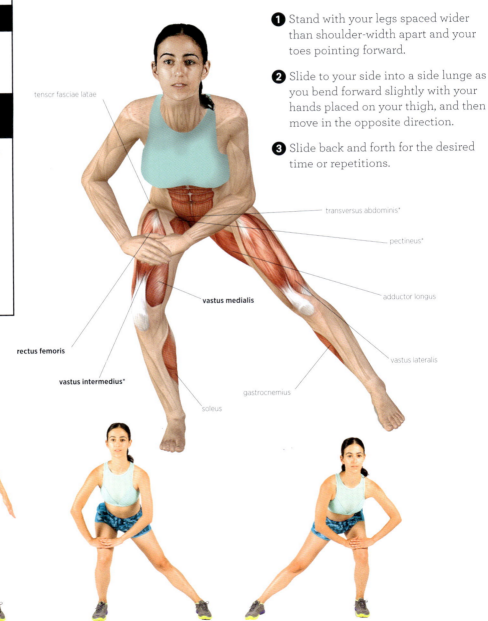

tensor fasciae latae

transversus abdominis*

pectineus*

adductor longus

vastus medialis

vastus lateralis

rectus femoris

vastus intermedius*

gastrocnemius

soleus

BEGINNER

8 reps, 5-sec hold

INTERMEDIATE

8 reps, 10 secs per leg

ADVANCED

15 reps, 10 secs per leg

BEST FOR

- Glutes
- Spine
- Hamstrings

FIND YOUR FORM

- Make the stretch long and smooth, and reach down only as far as you can comfortably extend. As you lower your torso, keep your back flat, and tuck your abdominals in toward your spine. Lengthen your spine as much as possible.
- Avoid bouncing as you reach your fingers toward your toes.

TOE TOUCHES

Moving through daily life requires quite a bit of bending, whether you are reaching down to pick up your child or retrieving your dropped car keys. The Forward Bend and its variations prepare you to do these everyday movements with ease and efficiency, and they also get you in shape for high-intensity activities like gymnastics and martial arts. Bending exercises can strengthen muscles and joints while helping you to become more flexible by stretching and opening tight areas of your body. The Forward Bend particularly targets the hamstrings muscles and the spine.

1 Stand tall with your arms at your sides.

2 Raise your arms toward the ceiling.

3 Exhale and bend forward from your hips, sweeping your arms to the sides with your palms facing the floor.

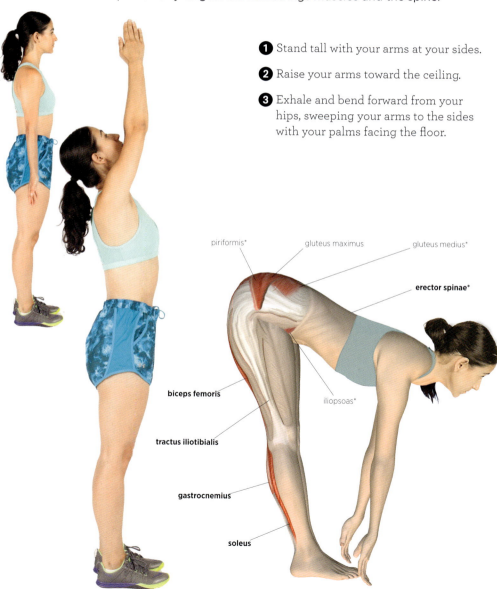

piriformis*

gluteus maximus

gluteus medius*

erector spinae*

biceps femoris

iliopsoas*

tractus iliotibialis

gastrocnemius

soleus

BEGINNER

Jog in place, 1 min

INTERMEDIATE

Jog in place, 90 secs

ADVANCED

Jog in place, 2 mins

BEST FOR

- Glutes
- Quads
- Hamstrings
- Calves

FIND YOUR FORM

- Build up speed as you go.
- Push off from your entire foot.
- Avoid pushing solely off your toes.

BUTT KICK

Doing the Butt Kick regularly will make those often-problematic hamstrings much stronger—which helps with so many types of exercise and sports. It should also give your cardiovascular system a mild workout.

1 Begin in a standing position, and then jog in place.

2 Kick your heels up high toward your buttocks.

3 Continue jogging in place, lifting your heels high, for the recommended time while increasing your speed as you go.

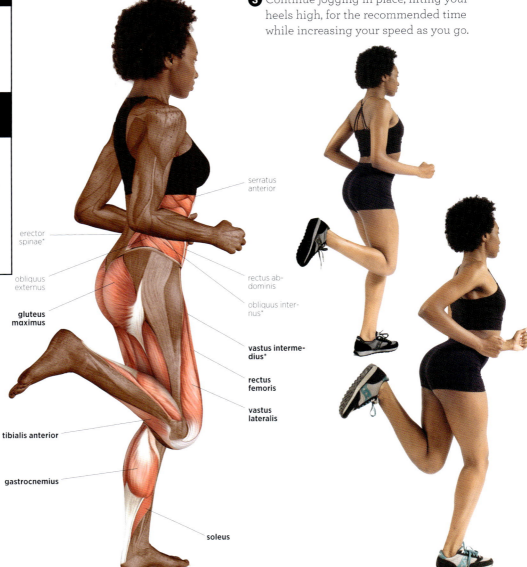

serratus anterior

erector spinae*

obliquus externus

gluteus maximus

rectus abdominis

obliquus internus*

vastus intermedius*

rectus femoris

vastus lateralis

tibialis anterior

gastrocnemius

soleus

1 MIN TARGETS

BEGINNER

Jog in place, 1 min

INTERMEDIATE

Jog in place, 90 secs

ADVANCED

Jog in place, 2 mins

BEST FOR

- Glutes
- Quads
- Hamstrings
- Calves

FIND YOUR FORM

- Keep the back long and upright. Keep the abs glued into the lower back to support the core.
- Do not let the shoulders hunch forward, or open too far behind you. Keep your abdominals engaged for proper alignment.

HIGH KNEES

When you bring your knee up past hip height you are engaging your core deeply, and also giving the lower back a stretch down through the hamstring. Alternating the knees up into the chest in this exercise will increase your balance, agility, and core strength.

1 Stand tall with your arms long at your sides.

2 Engage the core and the backs of your legs and lift the right knee high into the chest.

3 In one quick move, step the right leg down and bring the left leg up. Allow both legs to bend as you move through the exercise.

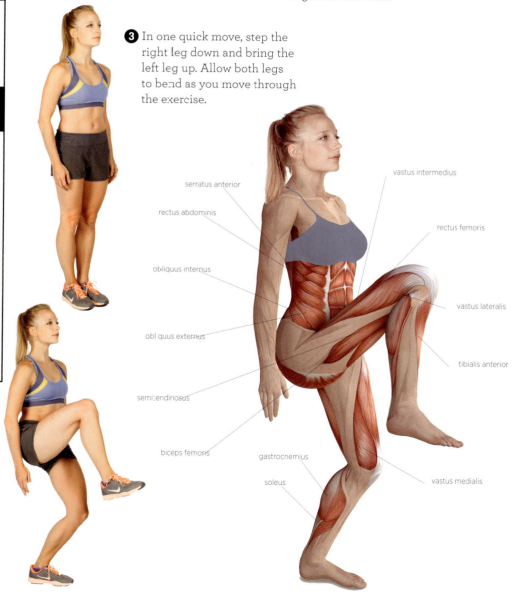

serratus anterior

rectus abdominis

obliquus internus

obliquus externus

semitendinosus

biceps femoris

gastrocnemius

soleus

vastus intermedius

rectus femoris

vastus lateralis

tibialis anterior

vastus medialis

1 MIN TARGETS

BEGINNER

20 reps per side

INTERMEDIATE

30 reps per side

ADVANCED

50 reps per leg

BEST FOR

- Glutes
- Quads
- Hamstrings
- Calves

FIND YOUR FORM

- Keep facing forward.
- When stepping over the bench, be sure to raise your leg, and then rotate your thigh outward—avoid just turning your torso to step over the bench.

The Lateral Step-Over is great exercise to help you improve lateral quickness and increase your agility. Perform it as a drill to really focus on your coordination, starting at half speed and, as the footwork becomes familiar, working up to moving as quickly as you can while maintaining good form. You can also vary the height and width of your obstacle—try setting up small cones or a low step to start out, eventually stepping over higher benches or steps.

1 Stand next to a step or flat bench.

2 Raise the knee of the leg closest to the bench and then lower your foot down to the floor on the opposite side of the bench.

3 Lift the opposite leg to meet the other, bringing your feet together.

4 Reverse the motion until you are standing with both feet together in the starting position. Repeat in a continuous motion for the desired time or reps.

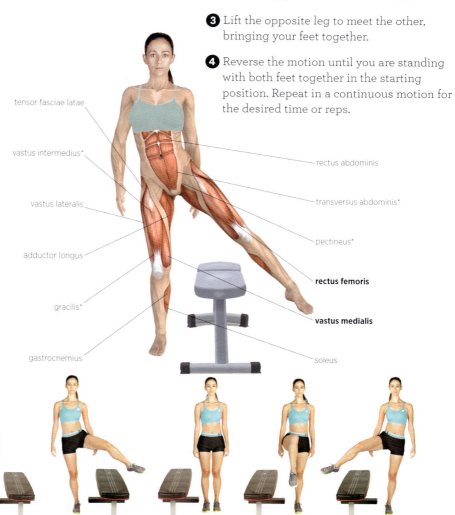

tensor fasciae latae

vastus intermedius*

vastus lateralis

adductor longus

gracilis*

gastrocnemius

rectus abdominis

transversus abdominis*

pectineus*

rectus femoris

vastus medialis

soleus

1 MIN TARGETS

BEGINNER
Skip in place, 1 min

INTERMEDIATE
Skip in place, 90 secs

ADVANCED
Skip in place, 2 mins

BEST FOR

• Shoulders
• Thighs
• Calves

FIND YOUR FORM

• Begin with the right rope. To judge the proper length, stand on the middle of the rope—the handles should extend to your armpits. To begin the exercise, hold the rope with your hands at about hip height with your elbows slightly bent. Keep your upper arms close to your sides as you swing the rope with your chest out and your shoulders back and down.

• Avoid jumping too high; keep your jumps small, and make sure to land on the balls of your feet

JUMP ROPE

Skipping, or jumping, rope, may be a schoolyard favorite, but like many a childhood activity, it is a high-energy exercise that really burns calories. Athletes, such as boxers, and military personnel are known for skipping rope as a training move, and it is an effective exercise to perform as a rest between other exercise sets to recover your heart rate.

❶ Stand with the jump rope in your hands, letting the rope hang behind your feet.

❷ Swing the rope around your body and jump over it. Keep your arms as straight as you can during the movement, and land with both feet together on the floor.

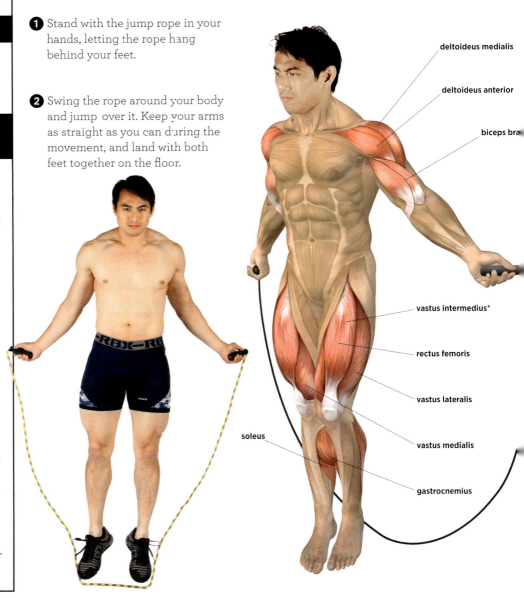

deltoideus medialis

deltoideus anterior

biceps bra

vastus intermedius*

rectus femoris

vastus lateralis

soleus

vastus medialis

gastrocnemius

BEGINNER

4 x 10 sec holds + rest

INTERMEDIATE

3 x 15 sec holds + rest

ADVANCED

2 x 30 sec holds

BEST FOR

- Adductors
- Hip flexors

FIND YOUR FORM

- Stretch until you reach a challenging position but without pain.
- Avoid placing too much weight on your knees.
- Don't allow your lower back to sink.

FROG STRADDLE

The Frog Straddle offers a deep stretch in your inner-thigh muscles. Using the weight of your body, you can direct this stretch to target different muscle groups.

1 Kneel on all fours.

2 Bend your elbows, shift your weight forward, and lower your elbows and forearms onto the floor.

3 Spread your knees apart, drawing your feet in slightly and putting some weight on them to take pressure off your knees.

4 Lower your legs and buttocks down to the floor and bring the soles of your feet together to deepen the stretch.

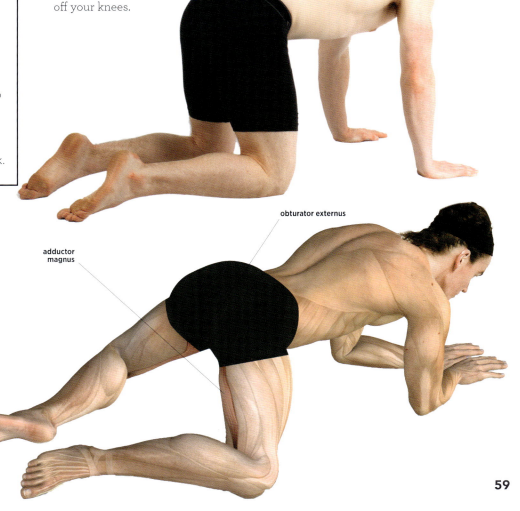

obturator externus

adductor magnus

1 MIN TARGETS

BEGINNER

15 reps per side

INTERMEDIATE

20 reps per side

ADVANCED

30 reps per side

BEST FOR

- Quads
- Hamstrings
- Glutes

FIND YOUR FORM

- Push through the working heel, keeping that foot planted.
- Avoid hyperextending your knee past your toes or moving faster than you can while still maintaining control.

STEP UP

As part of a strength and conditioning program, the Step Up effectively tones and sculpts your lower-body muscles, especially your quads, glutes, hip flexors, and hamstrings. It is also a great balance move for improving stability in your pelvis and legs, and adds a strong dose of cardio to a workout. Start with a step or box high enough that you must bend your knee to at least a 90-degree angle. Build up to higher boxes or benches as your strength and stamina improve.

1 Stand in front of a step or bench.

2 Step onto the bench with your right leg, making sure your foot is flat on the bench.

3 Lean forward slightly and push upward through the heel of your right foot, stepping up so that your left foot rests on the bench.

4 Step down with your right leg, and repeat the same sequence with your left leg. Continue stepping up and down, alternating sides.

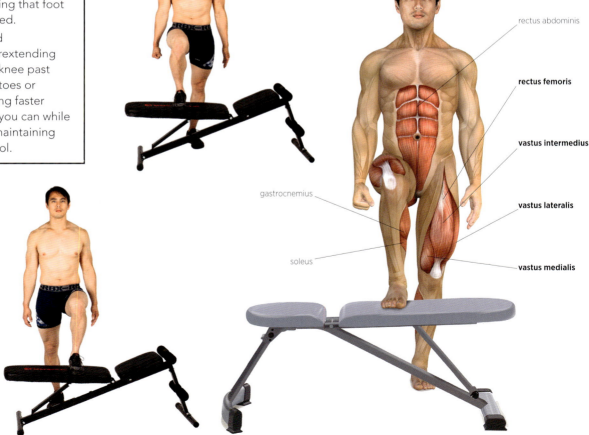

rectus abdominis

rectus femoris

vastus intermedius

vastus lateralis

vastus medialis

gastrocnemius

soleus

BEGINNER
4 x 10 sec holds + rest

INTERMEDIATE
3 x 15 sec holds + rest

ADVANCED
2 x 30 sec holds

BEST FOR

- Abdominals
- Hip flexors
- Chest
- Thighs
- Glutes
- Back
- Neck

FIND YOUR FORM

- Maintain strongly engaged lower abdominals.
- Keep your inner thighs active to maintain parallel legs.
- Keep your hips level.
- Avoid jamming your chin into your chest.
- Avoid letting your rib cage "pop" forward and upward.
- Avoid arching, and pushing into, your lower back while in the bridge.

BRIDGE

Bridge pose is a favorite of all kinds of exercise programs—because it opens up and strengthens so effectively. This is a great exercise for the upper body, while also putting your legs through their paces.

1 Lie on your back, with your pelvis and spine aligned but feeling natural and not pressed flat to the floor. Your legs should be bent with feet on the floor, and your knees aligned with your hips and feet. Your feet shouldn't be too far away from your buttocks, and firmly planted on the floor. Extend your arms along your sides, palms downward, and press your shoulders down your back to stabilize your shoulder blades.

2 Bend your knees as deeply as you can, squatting down until your hips are lower than your knees.

3 Curl your spine back toward the floor, starting with your cervical vertebrae and rolling down your thoracic vertebrae and farther down to your lumbar vertebrae.

4 Repeat for the recommended repetitions.

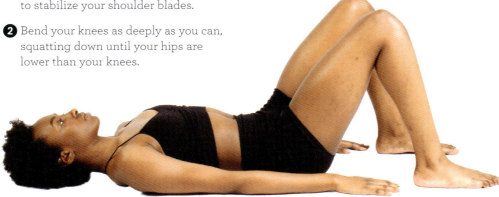

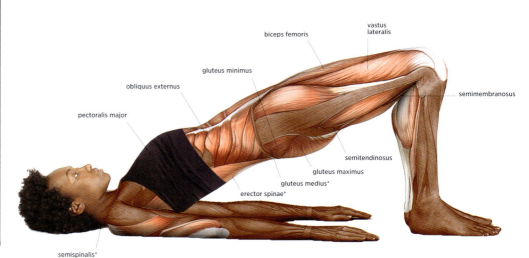

vastus lateralis

biceps femoris

gluteus minimus

obliquus externus

pectoralis major

semimembranosus

semitendinosus

gluteus maximus

gluteus medius*

erector spinae*

semispinalis*

1 MIN TARGETS

BEGINNER

4 x 10 sec holds + rest

INTERMEDIATE

3 x 15 sec holds + rest

ADVANCED

2 x 30 sec holds

BEST FOR

- Spine
- Abdominals
- Thighs
- Glutes

FIND YOUR FORM

- Engage your buttocks throughout.
- Keep your hips level at all times.
- Extend your leg out through your foot.
- Avoid arching your back.
- Avoid twisting or tilting your hips while lifting.

ONE-LEGGED BRIDGE

This Bridge Pose stretches your chest, spine, and thighs while strengthening your core and buttocks. It also eases stress by relieving tension in your back and shoulders.

1 Lie on your back with your arms out to your sides. Bend your knees and align your feet directly under your knees.

2 Exhale and press down through your feet to lift your buttocks off the floor. With your feet and thighs parallel, push your arms into the floor while extending through your fingertips.

3 Lengthen your neck away from your shoulders. Lift your hips higher so that your torso rises from the floor.

4 Straighten your right leg so that it is fully extended, forming a straight line from hip to toe.

5 Hold for the recommended time, return to the starting position, and then repeat on the opposite side.

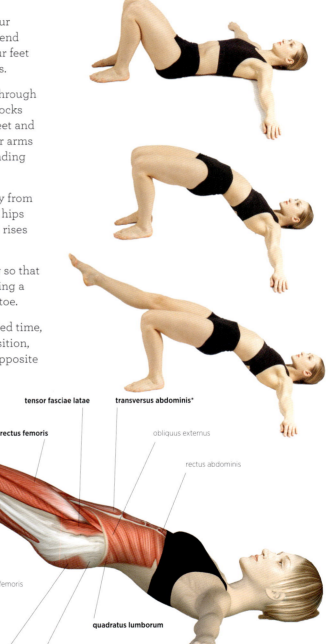

vastus lateralis

rectus femoris

tensor fasciae latae

transversus abdominis*

obliquus externus

rectus abdominis

biceps femoris

quadratus lumborum

gluteus maximus

gluteus medius*

BEGINNER
4 x 10 sec holds + rest

INTERMEDIATE
3 x 15 sec holds + rest

ADVANCED
2 x 30 sec holds

BEST FOR

- Quads
- Inner thighs
- Hamstrings

FIND YOUR FORM

- Keep the body in one line from the knees to the top of the head, on both the front and back sides of the body!
- Do not allow the thighs to grip, straining the quad muscles. Keep your muscles long and still

THIGH ROCK-BACK

These rock-backs focus the bulk of work into your quads, inner thighs, hamstrings, and glute muscles. By kneeling and isolating the knee joint to bend deeply, hinging the weight of your body back into space, behind your center plunge line, you engage all the muscles in your core and lower legs deeply!

❶ Kneel on top of a soft surface, with your knees slightly apart in a hip-width stance.

❷ Let your arms hang at the sides of your body.

❸ Lengthen your spine long, pull your abdominals in toward your lower back.

❹ Squeeze your butt muscles and hamstrings, and allow the weight of your body to lean back into the space behind.

❺ Squeeze the legs and core to bring you back up straight.

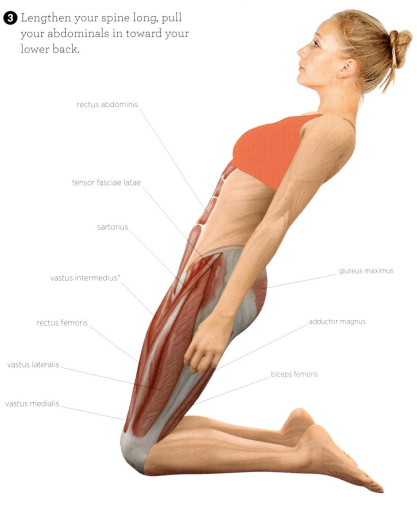

rectus abdominis

tensor fasciae latae

sartorius

vastus intermedius*

rectus femoris

vastus lateralis

vastus medialis

gluteus maximus

adductor magnus

biceps femoris

1 MIN TARGETS

BEGINNER
8 x 5 sec holds + rest

INTERMEDIATE
6 x 10 sec holds + rest

ADVANCED
4 x 30 sec holds

BEST FOR

- Quads
- Hamstrings
- Abs

FIND YOUR FORM

- Keep your torso facing forward and in line with your leg to help maintain your balance.
- Avoid sinking your neck into your shoulders.

KNEELING SIDE LIFT

Tone your outer thighs and outer core with this Pilates-inspired stretching exercise. Take care not to let your extended foot touch the floor until the movement is complete.

1 Begin by kneeling on the floor. Extend your right leg out to your side, keeping your left thigh aligned with your hips.

2 Place your hands behind your head, with your elbows pressed out to your sides.

3 Lift your right leg off the floor to hip height, as you bend your torso to your left.

4 Hold this pose for the recommended time, release the stretch, and repeat on the opposite side.

obliquus internus*

obliquus externus

rectus abdominis

tensor fasciae atae

vastus intermedius*

vastus lateralis

transversus abdominis*

iliopsoas*

rectus femoris

sartorius

SIDE KICK

Static Side Kicks, in which you push the leg out from the midline and then bring it back in, without moving any other part, are excellent for stabilizing the sides of the body. They also help with strengthening the core and enhancing balance.

1 Stand tall with your core engaged and the spine very long.

2 Reach the arms long at your sides and open the legs to shoulder width.

3 In one movement, swing the right leg open to the side and open the arms up wide to help keep you balanced. Flex the right foot.

4 Allow the weight of the leg to bring it back to starting, and then change sides.

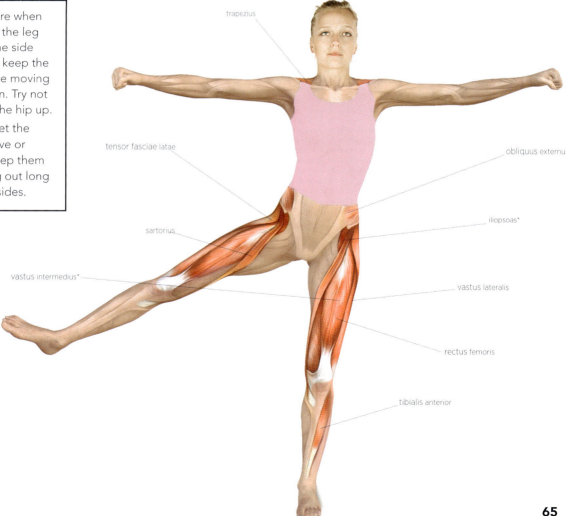

trapezius

tensor fasciae latae

obliquus externus

iliopsoas*

sartorius

vastus intermedius*

vastus lateralis

rectus femoris

tibialis anterior

1 MIN TARGETS

BEGINNER

2 x 20 sec holds + rest

INTERMEDIATE

3 x 15 sec holds + rest

ADVANCED

2 x 30 sec holds

BEST FOR

- Inner thighs
- Hamstrings
- Glutes
- Rib cage
- Hip flexors

FIND YOUR FORM

- Keep the turnout in your legs, and aim your toes straight up.
- Avoid lifting your hip bones off the floor.
- Don't allow your legs to turn inward.

WIDE ANGLE SEATED FORWARD BEND

Wide-Angle Seated Forward Bend is a challenging pose that opens your hips and groin muscles and lengthens your spine. For those who are limber enough to relax into this stretch, it is a restful posture offering a full-body stretch.

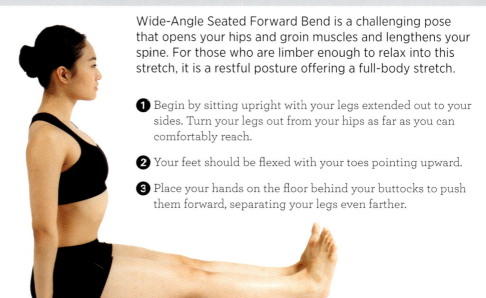

❶ Begin by sitting upright with your legs extended out to your sides. Turn your legs out from your hips as far as you can comfortably reach.

❷ Your feet should be flexed with your toes pointing upward.

❸ Place your hands on the floor behind your buttocks to push them forward, separating your legs even farther.

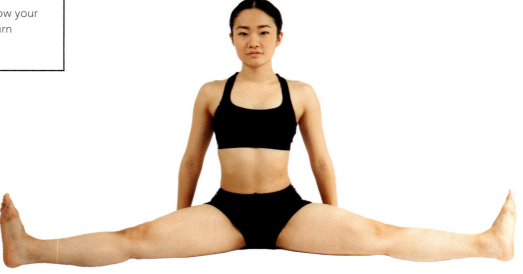

4 Press the backs of your thighs and sit bones into the floor.

5 Lift up through your torso and reach your hands to the floor in front of you.

6 Slowly walk your hands forward as you lower your torso toward the floor. Stretch as far as possible without rounding your back.

7 Hold for the recommended time, and then release the stretch.

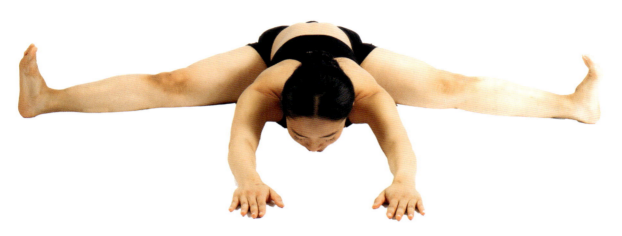

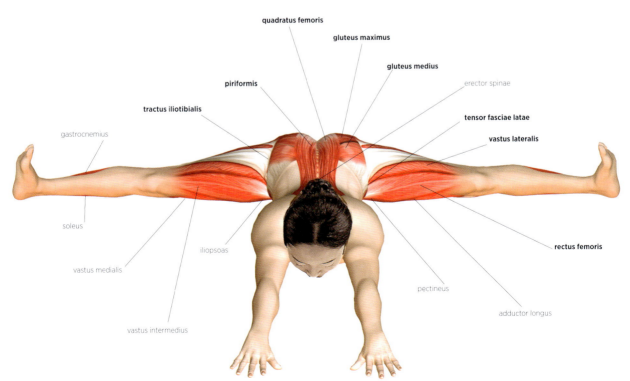

quadratus femoris

gluteus maximus

gluteus medius

piriformis

erector spinae

tractus iliotibialis

tensor fasciae latae

gastrocnemius

vastus lateralis

soleus

rectus femoris

iliopsoas

vastus medialis

pectineus

vastus intermedius

adductor longus

1 MIN TARGETS

BEGINNER

2 x 20 sec holds + rest

INTERMEDIATE

3 x 15 sec holds + rest

ADVANCED

2 x 30 sec holds

BEST FOR

• Spine
• Hips

FIND YOUR FORM

• Keep your knees soft.

• Hinge forward with your chest open and your back flat.

• Bend only as far forward as you can go while maintaining your flat back.

• Keep your hips lined up above your heels. (To this end, it helps to shift your weight onto the balls of your feet.)

WIDE LEGGED FORWARD BEND

Another very simple exercise that really delivers for your buttocks and legs. The Squat works your abdominals, too, which means that it helps to stabilize your core. Plus the pose promotes better balance.

2 Stand in the middle of your mat in Mountain Pose with your hands on your hips. Step or jump your feet so that they are parallel, 3 to 4 feet apart.

3 On an inhalation, lengthen your spine, lift your chest, and find a slight bend in your upper back, bringing your gaze up to the ceiling.

2 Exhaling, hinge forward from your hips until your palms are on the floor, with your fingers facing forward. Walk your hands back until your hands are in line with your heels. Bring the crown of your head toward the floor, lifting your shoulders toward your ears to make space for your neck.

3 Roll your right thigh counter-clockwise and your left thigh clockwise to find internal rotation in your legs. Firm your thighs, and lift your kneecaps up. Let your sitting bones move toward the ceiling as your tailbone draws down toward the floor. Hold for prescribed time

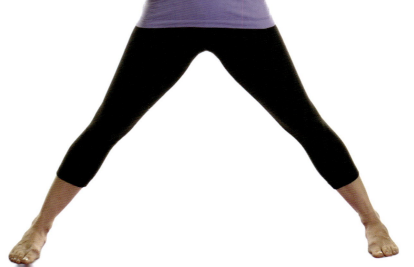

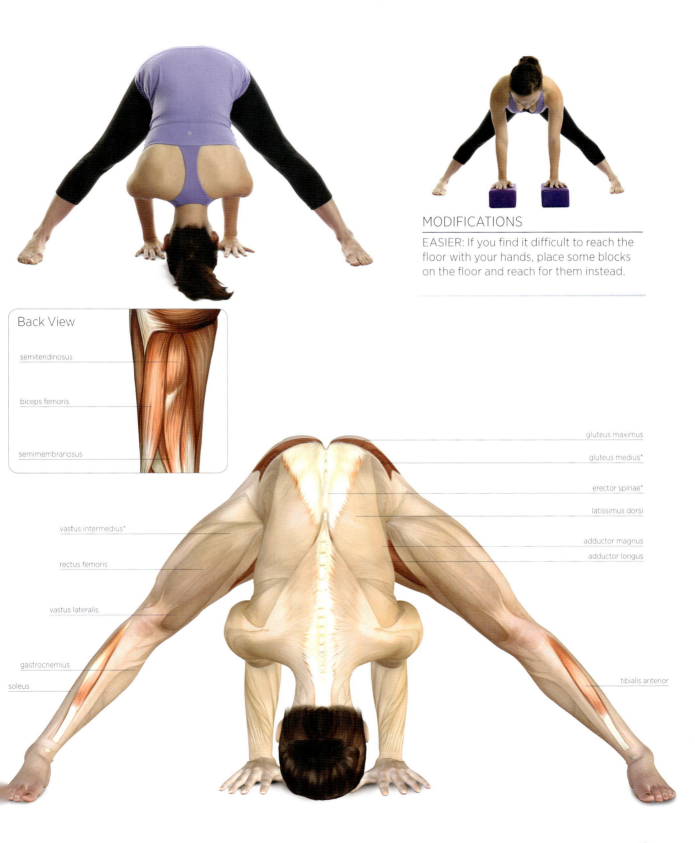

MODIFICATIONS

EASIER: If you find it difficult to reach the floor with your hands, place some blocks on the floor and reach for them instead.

Back View

semitendinosus

biceps femoris

semimembranosus

gluteus maximus

gluteus medius*

erector spinae*

latissimus dorsi

vastus intermedius*

adductor magnus

adductor longus

rectus femoris

vastus lateralis

gastrocnemius

soleus

tibialis anterior

1 MIN TARGETS

BEGINNER
4 x 10 sec holds + rest

INTERMEDIATE
3 x 15 sec holds + rest

ADVANCED
2 x 30 sec holds

BEST FOR

- Quads
- Hamstrings
- Glutes

FIND YOUR FORM

- Squat deep, and be sure to keep your thighs parallel to the floor.
- Avoid hyperextending your knees past your toes while squatting.

SINGLE LEG GLUTEAL LIFT

The Single-Leg Gluteal Lift develops tight, strong glutes while working many other major muscles. A key to safe success here is to use your abdominals to lift your body.

1 Lie on your back with your arms along your sides and legs bent with your feet directly under your knees. Extend your left leg upward, pointing through your foot.

2 Engage your abdominals to pop up to a one-legged, stable Bridge pose. Raise your body only as high as you can go while maintaining correct alignment.

3 Maintain this position, focusing on keeping your hips level, navel pressing to spine, and your raised leg extending from the hip joint.

4 Lower your body back down to the floor, keeping your left leg extended.

5 Repeat the bridge, with the same leg raised, for the recommended repetitions. Switch legs and repeat on the opposite side for the recommended repetitions.

soleus

gastrocnemius

semimembranosus

biceps femoris

semitendinosus

vastus lateralis

rectus femoris

vastus intermedius*

tensor fasciae latae

transversus abdominis*

obliquus internus*

obliquus externus

sartorius

gluteus maximus

latissimus dorsi

70

HALF SQUAT WITH ARMS RAISED

This stretch, known as Chair Pose in the discipline of yoga, will increase your strength, balance, and stability while activating just about every muscle in your body. It calls for you to sustain an unsupported sitting position as you extend your arms and engage the muscles in your shoulders and upper back.

1 Stand with your feet together and arms by your sides.

2 Inhale as you reach your arms out to your sides, and continue lifting until you are standing with your arms above your head. Your hands should be shoulder-width apart.

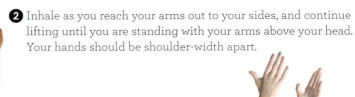

3 Straighten your arms, and rotate your shoulders externally open so that the palms of your hands face each other, spreading up through your fingertips.

4 Exhale, and bend your knees. Both ankles, inner thighs, and knees should be touching. Bring your weight onto your heels, shift your hips back, and draw your knees right above your ankles

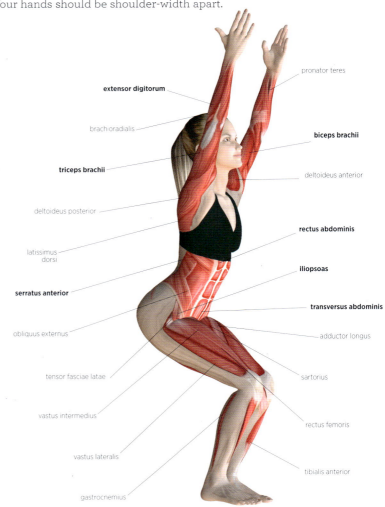

extensor digitorum

brachioradialis

triceps brachii

deltoideus posterior

latissimus dorsi

serratus anterior

obliquus externus

tensor fasciae latae

vastus intermedius

vastus lateralis

gastrocnemius

pronator teres

biceps brachii

deltoideus anterior

rectus abdominis

iliopsoas

transversus abdominis

adductor longus

sartorius

rectus femoris

tibialis anterior

1 MIN TARGETS

BEGINNER

4 x 10 sec holds + rest

INTERMEDIATE

3 x 15 sec holds + rest

ADVANCED

2 x 30 sec holds

BEST FOR

• Quads
• Hamstrings
• Core

FIND YOUR FORM

• Keep your back flat by pulling in the abdominals deeply in toward the lower back.

• Do not position the knees in or out further than a 90-degree angle. Square alignment is key in this set of movements.

FIRE HYDRANT

This core-exercise variation can be found in almost all abdominal-focused workouts like yoga, Pilates, ballet barre, and calisthenics. The focus is on keeping the core stabilized between two hands and one leg, while you lift and lower the other leg to the side, working the inner and outer muscles of the hip and glutes.

1 Come to balance on your hands and knees (quadruped position).

2 Come to balance on your hands and knees (quadruped position).

3 Lift your right leg out to the side, keeping the knee bent and your chest facing the ground.

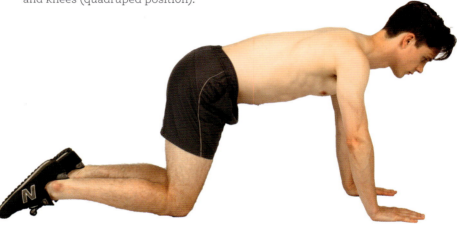

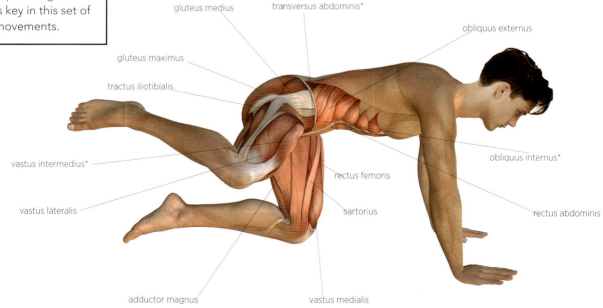

gluteus medius
transversus abdominis*
obliquus externus
gluteus maximus
tractus iliotibialis
obliquus internus*
vastus intermedius*
rectus femoris
vastus lateralis
sartorius
rectus abdominis
adductor magnus
vastus medialis

1 MIN TARGETS

BEGINNER

4 x 10 beats + rest

INTERMEDIATE

3 x 20 beats

ADVANCED

2 x 30 beats

BEST FOR

• Adductors
• Glutes

FIND YOUR FORM

• Stabilize your shoulder girdle.

• Keep your hips firmly pressed into the floor as you press your navel toward your spine.

• Stretch your legs fully without locking your knees.

• Avoid lifting your legs so high that you feel tension in your lower back.

• Avoid altering the slightly turned-out position of your legs.

EXTENSION HEEL BEATS

This exercise is especially effective for your glutes and inner-thigh adductors, but it also works much of your core and upper legs. As with all exercises performed in a prone position, keep your abdominals fully engaged.

1 Lie on your stomach, resting your forehead on the back of your stacked hands. Slightly rotate your legs from the hip joints outward and press the inner sides of your legs and your heels together.

2 Fully engage your glutes. Slightly lift your extended legs up from the floor.

3 With your feet fairly pointed, lightly beat your heels together for the recommended number of times.

4 Flex your feet (that is, not pointed), and move your legs to hip-distance apart. Hold for the recommended time.

5 Now stretch out your feet again and press your legs and heels together to begin another set of heel beats. Repeat for the recommended repetitions.

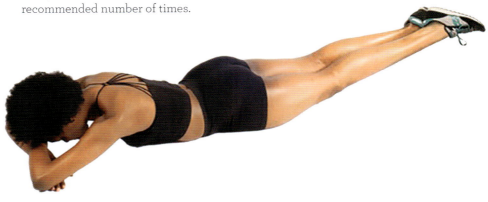

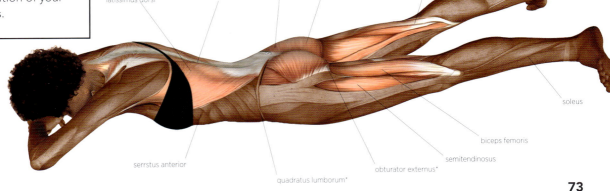

gluteus maximus

semimembranosus

gluteus medius*

erector spinae*

latissimus dorsi

soleus

biceps femoris

semitendinosus

serrstus anterior

obturator externus*

quadratus lumborum*

CORE

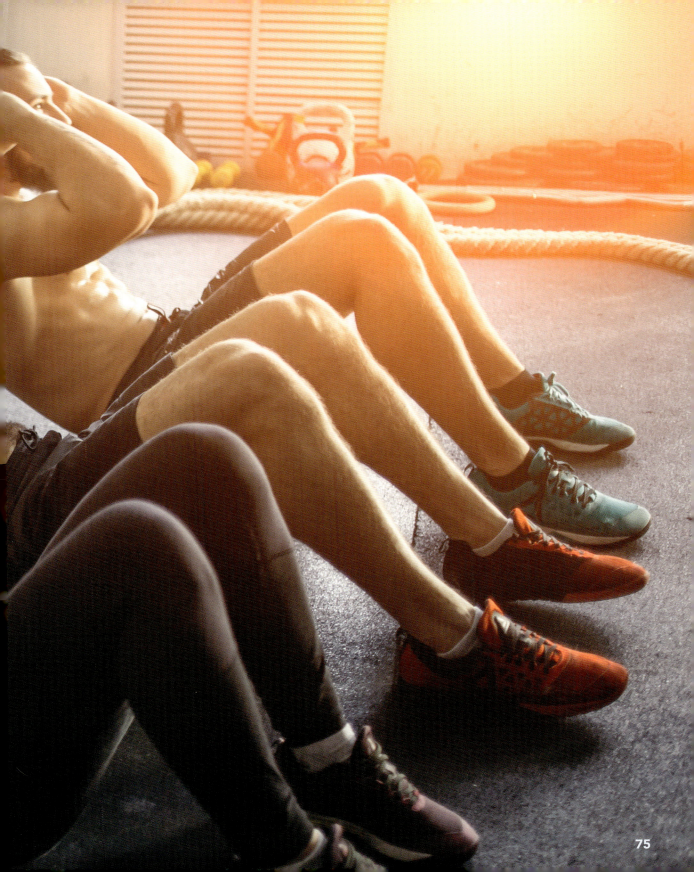

1 MIN TARGETS

BEGINNER
15 reps

INTERMEDIATE
20 reps

ADVANCED
40 reps

BEST FOR

- Core
- Thighs
- Back

FIND YOUR FORM

- Squat deep, and be sure to keep your thighs parallel to the floor.
- Avoid hyperextending your knees past your toes while squatting.

SIT-UP

The Sit-Up is a classic move that you are sure to find in just about all workout routines. Athletes and performers alike utilize Sit-Ups for their ability to stabilize and strengthen the upper body. The Sit-Up is a movement that works every inch of the core—from our multi-layered abdominals through to the backs of our bodies. Stabilizing the muscle groups that support our spine betters the total movement of our entire body, both upper and lower.

1 Lie down on your back and bring your feet in, along the floor, about 2 feet (60 cm) from your hips.

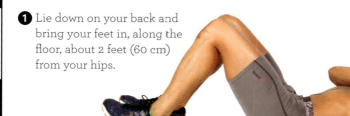

2 Stack your hands across the chest onto the tops of your shoulders.

3 Engage your abs, tuck your chin into your chest, and curl your body up until your torso comes off the floor and is at a right angle to the floor.

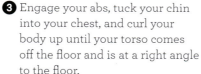

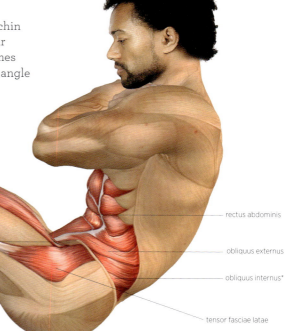

rectus femoris

tibialis anterior

iliopsoas*

rectus abdominis

obliquus externus

obliquus internus*

tensor fasciae latae

BEGINNER
15 reps

INTERMEDIATE
20 reps

ADVANCED
40 reps

BEST FOR

• Core
• Spine

FIND YOUR FORM

• Lead from your belly button, keeping your back straight.
• Avoid overusing your neck or arching your back to lift your torso.

BENT-KNEE ALTERNATING SIT-UP

The Alternating Sit-Up is an advanced variant on the classic Sit-Up. In addition to increasing the strength of the rectus abdominis and other core muscles, it focuses more intensely on the obliques. As such it is a key foundation exercise for abdominal and core strength.

1 Lie on your back with your legs slightly bent and your hands behind your head, elbows flat on the floor.

2 Push through your heels for support and raise your trunk off the ground by contracting your abdominal muscles.

3 As you rise, rotate to the right so your right elbow touches your right knee, and contract your oblique muscles.

4 Lower your back to the floor. Repeat the sit-up, this time rotating to the other side. Repeat as prescribed.

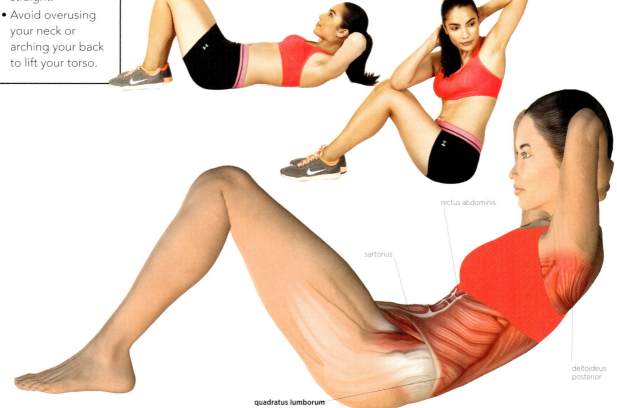

rectus abdominis

sartorius

deltoideus posterior

quadratus lumborum

1 MIN TARGETS

BEGINNER
10 reps

INTERMEDIATE
20 reps

ADVANCED
40 reps

BEST FOR

• Core
• Back
• Abs

FIND YOUR FORM

• Keep your lower back long on the floor and try not to arch your spine away from the ground under you.

• Avoid crunching the neck into your chest. You want to keep the neck long even if you cannot bring your body far up off the floor.

CRUNCH

You can find the Basic Crunch mixed in alongside many other Sit-Up type workouts. Performing a crunch is, essentially, the beginning part of the full Sit-Up. With the crunch, you do not bring your full torso up into flexion. Instead, you squeeze the abs into the lower back, keeping the front and back sides of the body long and strong against the floor. This shortening of the abdominal wall deeply strengthens the many layers that make up our cores.

1 Lie down on your back and bring your feet in, along the floor, about 2 feet (60 cm) from your hips.

2 Stack your hands behind the lower part of your head.

3 Engage your abs, tuck your chin into your chest, and curl your body up just until your upper back comes off the floor.

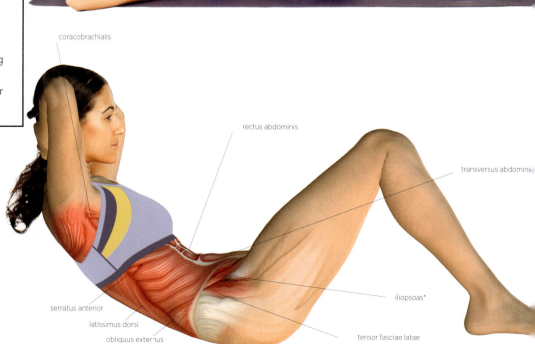

coracobrachialis

rectus abdominis

transversus abdominis

serratus anterior

latissimus dorsi

obliquus externus

iliopsoas*

tensor fasciae latae

BEGINNER
10 reps

INTERMEDIATE
20 reps

ADVANCED
40 reps

BEST FOR

• Core

FIND YOUR FORM

• Lift with your abdominals rather than your neck or back.
• Avoid using excessive momentum.

REVERSE CRUNCH

Reverse Crunch is highly effective for isolating the lowest portion of the rectus abdominis, where most abdominal fat tends to be stored. Less is more with this exercise: your movements should be small but focused.

1 Lie on your back with your arms at your sides and your legs bent at a 90-degree angle with your feet off the floor.

2 Lift your buttocks a few inches off the mat as you bring your knees toward your chest.

3 Lower in a controlled manner.

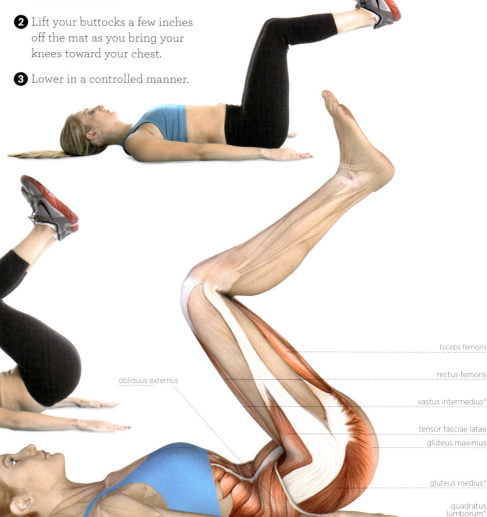

biceps femoris

rectus femoris

vastus intermedius*

tensor fasciae latae

gluteus maximus

gluteus medius*

quadratus lumborum*

obliquus externus

1 MIN TARGETS

BEGINNER
10 reps

INTERMEDIATE
20 reps

ADVANCED
40 reps

BEST FOR

- Abs
- Obliques
- Lower back

FIND YOUR FORM

- As you reach, pull in using your midsection.
- Avoid overusing your neck and/or back muscles.

PENGUIN CRUNCH

Penguin Crunch, also called Penguin Heel Reach, targets your oblique muscles. Because it incorporates lateral movement of the abdominals, it is a great exercise to prepare you for any sport that requires rotational movement, such as swimming or diving.

1 Begin on your back, with your head elevated and your arms at your sides and raised off the floor.

2 Reach forward in a stabbing motion with one hand, and then pull back.

3 Lower, and then repeat with the other hand. Repeat as prescribed.

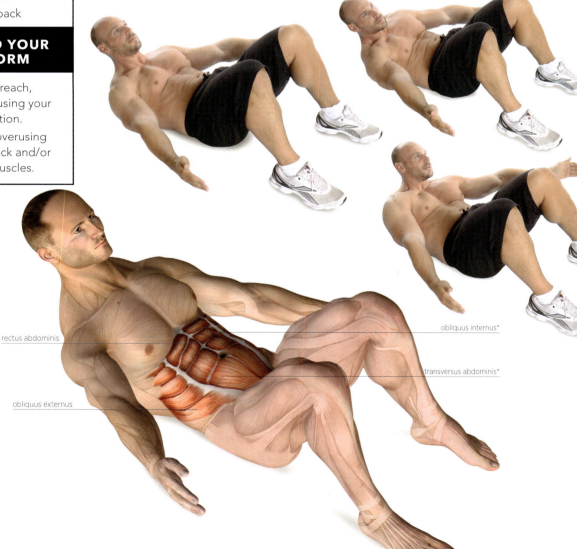

rectus abdominis

obliquus externus

obliquus internus*

transversus abdominis*

1 MIN TARGETS

BEGINNER

10 kicks

INTERMEDIATE

30 kicks

ADVANCED

50 kicks

BEST FOR

- Abs
- Obliques

FIND YOUR FORM

- Raise your elbow and opposite knee equally, so that they meet in the middle.
- Avoid raising your lower back off the floor.

BICYCLE CRUNCH

Bicycle Crunch is particularly effective for strengthening and toning your upper abdominals as well as your oblique muscles. Although you may be tempted to "cycle" quickly, perform each crunch smoothly and with control for best results.

1 Lie on your back with fingers at your ears, your elbows flared outward and your legs bent to form a 90-degree angle.

2 Begin to lift your shoulders and upper torso off the floor as your raise your right elbow diagonally. At the same time, bring your left knee toward your elbow and extend your right leg diagonally forward— until your right elbow and left knee meet.

3 Lower, and then repeat on the other side. Alternating, repeat as prescribed.

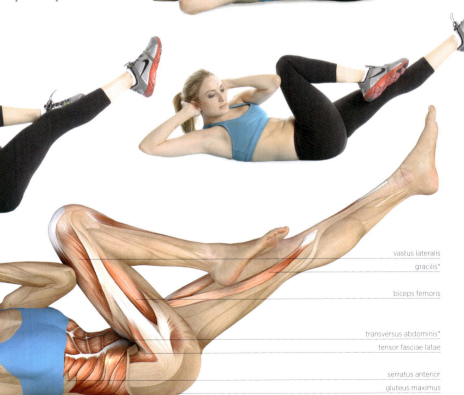

vastus lateralis

gracilis*

biceps femoris

transversus abdominis*

tensor fasciae latae

serratus anterior

gluteus maximus

biceps brachii

triceps brachii

1 MIN TARGETS

BEGINNER
15 reps

INTERMEDIATE
20 reps

ADVANCED
40 reps

BEST FOR

- Quads
- Hamstrings
- Glutes

FIND YOUR FORM

- Keep your arms and legs extended
- Lower your upper back just as slowly as you raised it.
- Press your legs together as if they were a single leg.
- Avoid using your lower-back muscles to drive the movement.

VERTICAL LEG CRUNCH

When carrying out Vertical Leg Crunch, you should feel a strong sense that your abs are not just getting stronger but becoming streamlined and defined, too. With your legs up, your abdominals do almost all the work. Keep your movement smooth as you lower yourself to the floor, so that your core stays active throughout all stages of the exercise.

1 Lie on your back, with your arms extended behind your head and your legs extended in front of you so that your body forms one straight line.

2 Bring your arms over your head so they are reaching straight upward, your hands directly above your shoulders and your arms forming a 90-degree angle with the floor. Raise your legs until they are parallel to your arms.

3 Using your abdominals to drive the movement, lift your shoulders off the floor, reaching your extended fingers towards your toes.

4 Lower and repeat as prescribed.

rectus femoris

biceps femoris

vastus intermedius*

tensor fasciae latae

obliquus externus

gluteus maximus

gluteus medius*

quadratus lumborum*

BEGINNER

6 reps, 5 sec hold

INTERMEDIATE

10 reps, 5 sec hold

ADVANCED

20 reps, 5 sec hold

BEST FOR

• Inner thighs

FIND YOUR FORM

• Apply gentle pressure between your elbows and your knees, encouraging your knees to open farther and deepening the inner-thigh stretch.

• Lengthen your spine, keeping your back straight.

• Broaden across your collarbones.

• Avoid rounding your shoulders forward.

V-UP

The challenging V-Up targets both your upper and lower rectus abdominis, as it moves through its entire range of motion. Performing V-Ups is also an efficient way to strengthen your lower-back muscles and tighten your quads.

❶ Lie on your back with your legs straight and your arms extended behind your head.

❷ Simultaneously raise your arms and legs so that your fingertips are nearly touching your feet, while maintaining a flat back.

❸ Lower and repeat as prescribed.

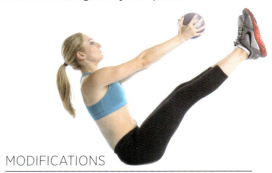

MODIFICATIONS

HARDER: Grasp a medicine ball in your hands, keeping it in place throughout the exercise.

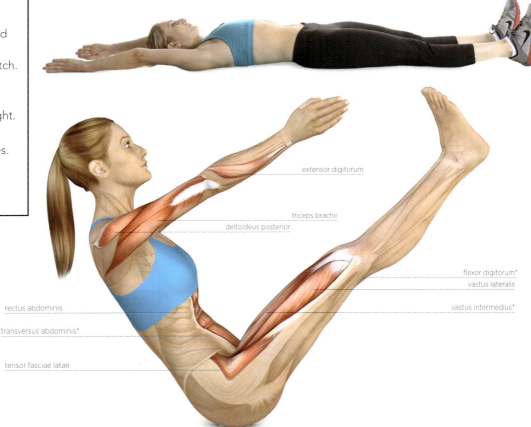

extensor digitorum

triceps brachii

deltoideus posterior

flexor digitorum*

vastus lateralis

vastus intermedius*

rectus abdominis

transversus abdominis*

tensor fasciae latae

1 MIN TARGETS

BEGINNER

6 reps, 5 sec hold

INTERMEDIATE

10 reps, 5 sec hold

ADVANCED

20 reps, 5 sec hold

BEST FOR

- Abdominals
- Thighs
- Hip flexors

FIND YOUR FORM

- Keep your neck stretched out.
- Maintain a tight core and a level pelvis.
- When balancing, your arms should be parallel to your extended leg.
- Avoid arching your back or rolling your shoulders forward.
- Avoid relying on momentum to propel you up or down.
- Avoid allowing your stomach to bulge outward.

SINGLE-LEG V-UP

Regular practice of Single-Leg V-Up will make your abdominal muscles stronger, which it turn makes the exercise's upward motion smoother and easier. This is a great way to prepare your core muscles for all kinds of workouts.

1 Lie on your back, with your arms extended over your head, hovering just above the floor behind you, palms up. Bend your knees and press them together. Anchor your feet into the floor.

2 Slowly and with control, extend your right leg, straightening it from your hip and out through your foot.

3 Initiating the movement from your lower abdomen, raise your torso to form a 45-degree angle with the floor as you bring your arms up and over your head to reach forward.

4 With control, curl your spine down to the floor as you bring your arms up overhead and behind you again, keeping your knees pressed together.

5 Repeat for the recommended repetitions. Repeat on the opposite side.

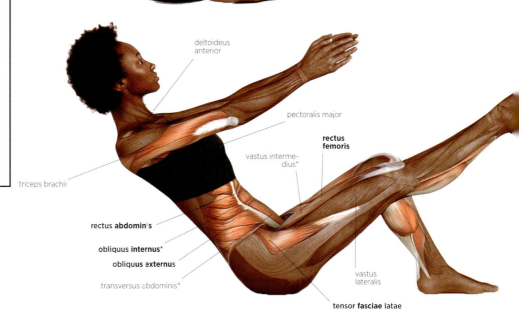

deltoideus anterior

pectoralis major

rectus femoris

vastus interme-dius*

triceps brachii

rectus **abdominis**

obliquus **internus***

obliquus **externus**

transversus abdominis*

vastus lateralis

tensor **fasciae** latae

1 MIN TARGETS

BEGINNER
4 x 10 sec holds + rest

INTERMEDIATE
3 x 15 sec holds + rest

ADVANCED
2 x 30 sec holds

BEST FOR

- Calves
- Core
- Achilles tendon

FIND YOUR FORM

- Keep your body in a straight line throughout the exercise.
- Avoid bending the knee of your supporting leg.

The aim of the Raised-leg pike is to build core strength, but it also deeply stretches your calves and Achilles tendon.

1 Begin by assuming a standard plank, or push-up, position.

2 Draw your right knee into your chest while leaning forward and flexing your foot. Keep your left foot flexed and balance on your toes.

3 Extend your left leg through the heel and rock your body back, shifting your weight into your left foot.

4 Keeping your spine aligned, straighten and extend your right leg toward the ceiling.

5 Hold for the recommended time, release the stretch, and then repeat on the opposite side.

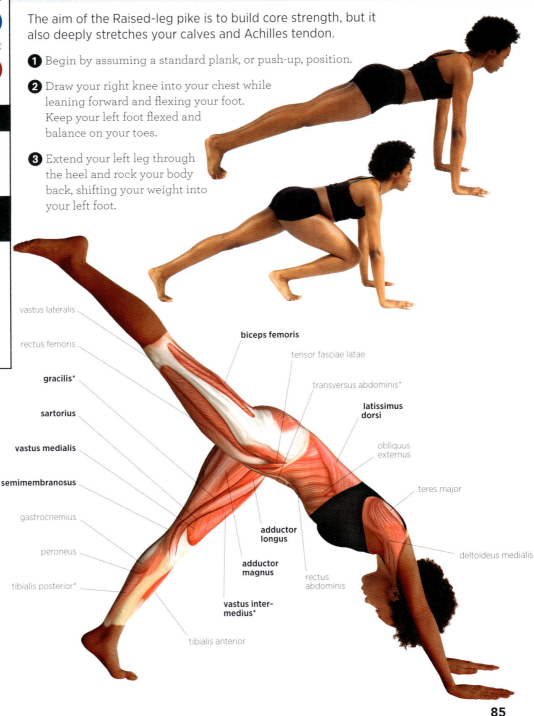

vastus lateralis

rectus femoris

gracilis*

sartorius

vastus medialis

semimembranosus

gastrocnemius

peroneus

tibialis posterior*

biceps femoris

tensor fasciae latae

transversus abdominis*

latissimus dorsi

obliquus externus

teres major

adductor longus

adductor magnus

rectus abdominis

deltoideus medialis

vastus inter-medius*

tibialis anterior

1 MIN TARGETS

BEGINNER

4 x 10 sec holds + rest

INTERMEDIATE

3 x 15 sec holds + rest

ADVANCED

2 x 30 sec holds

BEST FOR

- Quads
- Hamstrings
- Glutes

FIND YOUR FORM

- Fully engage your abs to keep your body in a stable line from feet to shoulders.
- Don't allow your hips to sag.

SWISS BALL BRIDGE

The Swiss Ball Bridge is low-intensity move that packs a lot of punch, effectively toning and strengthening your abdominals and glutes. You can amp up this basic move by adding leg lifts and curls to further increase its benefits.

1 Lie face-up on the floor with your arms at your sides and your lower legs resting on the Swiss ball.

2 Press your palms into the floor and engage your abdominal muscles as you lift your upper body off the floor. Your body should form a diagonal line. If desired, hold for a few seconds.

3 Slowly and with control, lower down to the starting position. Repeat for the desired repetitions.

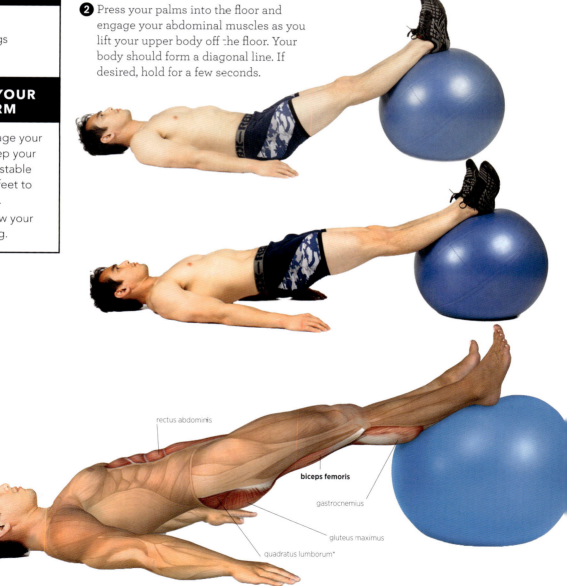

rectus abdominis

biceps femoris

gastrocnemius

gluteus maximus

quadratus lumborum*

BEGINNER

20 reps per side

INTERMEDIATE

30 reps per side

ADVANCED

50 reps per side

BEST FOR

• Spine
• Hip flexors
• Abdominals

FIND YOUR FORM

• Place your outside hand on the ankle of your bent leg, and your inside hand on your bent knee.

• Lift the top of your sternum forward.

• Avoid allowing your lower-back to rise off the floor.

• Use your abdominals to stabilize your core while switching legs.

ABDOMINAL KICK

When your hip flexors are tight, they pull on your lower spine, which can cause lower-back pain. Exercises like the reclining Abdominal Kick are a great way to keep your hip flexors limber, strengthen your core, and reduce tension in the lower vertebrae of your spine.

1 Lie supine on the floor with your knees bent.

2 Pull your right knee toward your chest and straighten your left leg, raising it about 45 degrees from the floor.

3 Place your right hand on your right ankle, and your left hand on your right knee to maintain proper alignment of your leg.

4 Alternate straightening and bending your legs, switching your hand placement at the same time.

5 Repeat for the recommended repetitions.

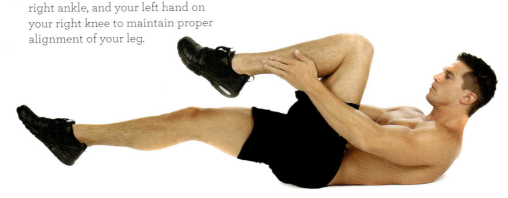

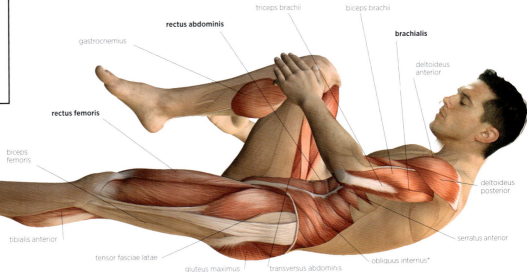

triceps brachii

biceps brachii

rectus abdominis

brachialis

gastrocnemius

deltoideus anterior

rectus femoris

biceps femoris

deltoideus posterior

serratus anterior

tibialis anterior

tensor fasciae latae

gluteus maximus

transversus abdominis

obliquus internus*

1 MIN TARGETS

BEGINNER

15 reps per side

INTERMEDIATE

25 reps per side

ADVANCED

40 reps per side

BEST FOR

- Abdominals
- Back
- Thighs

FIND YOUR FORM

- Keep your core muscles engaged and active.
- Stabilize your shoulders by pressing your shoulder blades down your back.
- Keep your buttocks firmly planted into the floor.
- Keep your legs lengthened.
- Avoid pulling your shoulders forward while grasping your leg.
- Avoid bending your knees.

SCISSORS

In Scissors, your legs are like scissor blades and your core like the handles. Keeping your handles stab e frees your blades to cut through the air precisely. This is a great way to build up your core.

❶ Lie on your back, with your pelvis lengthened along the floor but not jammed right into it. Place your arms along your sides, and fold your knees in toward your chest.

❷ Curl your head and neck off the floor, extending your legs to the ceiling one at a time. Both buttocks should remain anchored to the floor throughout the exercise.

❸ Extend both arms toward your left leg so you can grasp it with both hands while the leg remains straight. At the same time, lower your right leg halfway to the floor.

❹ Start to switch legs by reaching both of them up to the ceiling so that they cross each other in midair.

❺ Take hold of your extended right leg, and lower your left leg halfway to the floor.

❻ Alternate legs for the recommended repetitions.

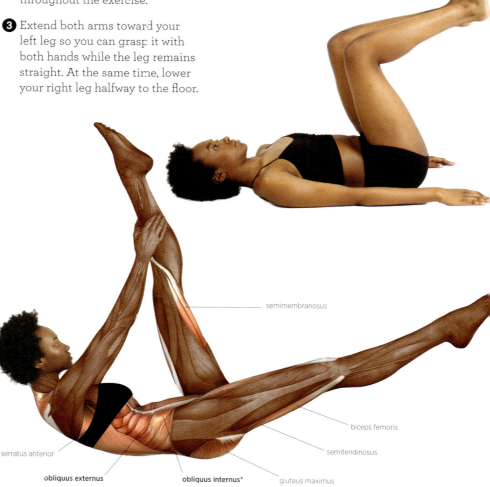

semimembranosus

biceps femoris

semitendinosus

serratus anterior

obliquus externus

obliquus internus*

gluteus maximus

BEGINNER

4 x 10 sec holds + rest

INTERMEDIATE

3 x 15 sec holds + rest

ADVANCED

2 x 30 sec holds

BEST FOR

- Glutes
- Back
- Abs

FIND YOUR FORM

- Apply gentle pressure between your elbows and your knees, encouraging your knees to open farther and deepening the inner-thigh stretch.
- Lengthen your spine, keeping your back straight.
- Broaden across your collarbones.
- Avoid rounding your shoulders forward.

BRIDGE WITH LEG LIFT

An excellent addition to the classic Bridge (see page 61), this exercise works the abdominals, back, and buttocks. It also improves balance. It can be simplified by decreasing the range of motion—just raise your foot slightly off the floor. If necessary, prop yourself up with your hands beneath your hips once in the bridge position.

1 Lie on the floor, your arms by your sides and fingers lengthened toward your feet. Your knees should be bent, with your feet flat on the floor.

2 Lift your hips and spine off the floor, creating one long line from your knees to your shoulders. Keep your weight over your feet.

3 Keeping your legs bent, bring your left knee toward your chest then lower it until your toe touches the mat. Bring your left knee toward your chest again. Lower leg to the floor.

4 Repeat the exercise with your right leg. Repeat as prescribed.

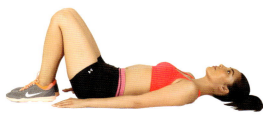

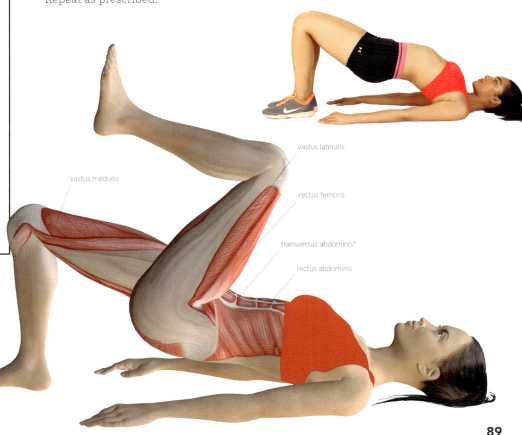

vastus lateralis

vastus medialis

rectus femoris

transversus abdominis*

rectus abdominis

1 MIN TARGETS

BEGINNER
10 reps

INTERMEDIATE
20 reps

ADVANCED
40 reps

BEST FOR

- Abdominals
- Obliques
- Lower Back

FIND YOUR FORM

- Maintain a precise and short range of motion.
- Keep the back straight and abs taut.
- Avoid using the neck to rise.
- Avoid bouncy and speedy repetitions.
- Avoid twisting the shoulders or back as you raise your torso.

ALTERNATING CRUNCH

The Alternating Crunch is an advanced version of the Crunch (see pages 78). It targets the obliques, in addition to the rectus abdominis. As with the Alternating Sit-Up, it is an exercise upon which the foundations of abdominal and core strength are built.

1 Begin by lying down on your back with your legs bent and your palms placed behind your head, elbows flared outward.

2 Raise your head and shoulders off the ground while contracting your trunk toward your waist.

3 From this half-sitting position, rotate your torso to bring your left elbow toward your right knee.

4 Lower your head and shoulders back to the floor then raise them again, this time bringing your right elbow toward your left knee. Repeat as prescribed.

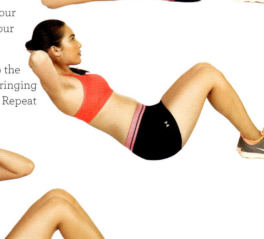

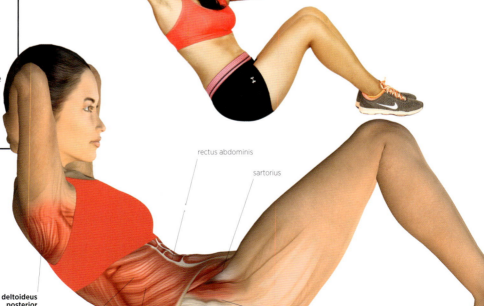

rectus abdominis

sartorius

deltoideus posterior

obliquus externus

obliquus internus*

tensor fasciate latae

90

BEGINNER
10 reps

INTERMEDIATE
20 reps

ADVANCED
40 reps

BEST FOR

- Abdominals
- Obliques
- Lower Back

FIND YOUR FORM

- To keep your abdominals fully engaged, be sure to keep moving smoothly with control, without pausing between repetitions.
- Avoid holding your breath.

SEATED RUSSIAN TWIST

The Russian Twist works your abdominals and obliques with its torso-rotating motion. Regularly performing this exercise or its variations increases abdominal endurance and builds explosiveness in the upper torso, which may help boost your performance in sports such as swimming, baseball, hockey, golf, lacrosse, and boxing.

1 Sit with your knees bent and your feet flat on the floor. Lift up through your torso. Raise your arms parallel to the floor so that your hands are outstretched above your knees.

2 Rotate your upper body to the right, reaching toward the floor with your hands.

3 Pass through the center and rotate to the left. Without stopping, continue moving with control from side to side.

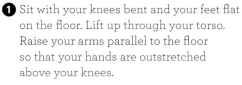

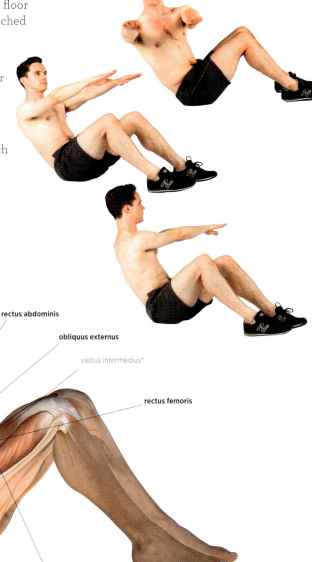

rectus abdominis

obliquus externus

vastus intermedius*

rectus femoris

latissimus dorsi

obliquus internus*

transversus abdominis*

iliopsoas*

tensor fasciae latae

vastus lateralis

1 MIN TARGETS

BEGINNER

30 reps

INTERMEDIATE

40 reps

ADVANCED

60 reps

BEST FOR

- Triceps
- Shoulders
- Core

FIND YOUR FORM

- Remain as stable as possible on top of the ball.
- Keep your fingers active and outstretched.
- Avoid allowing one or both feet to lift off the floor

SWISS BALL PRONE ROW

Swiss Ball Prone Row is an advanced exercise that challenges your rotator cuffs and upper back. It also effectively works your core. This exercise is best preceded by a thorough warm-up to loosen your shoulder girdle.

1 Begin facedown on top of a fitness ball, with your torso supported. Balance on your toes, with your legs separated for stability.

2 Bend your arms to form 90-degree angles, with your upper arms parallel to the floor.

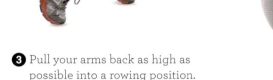

3 Pull your arms back as high as possible into a rowing position.

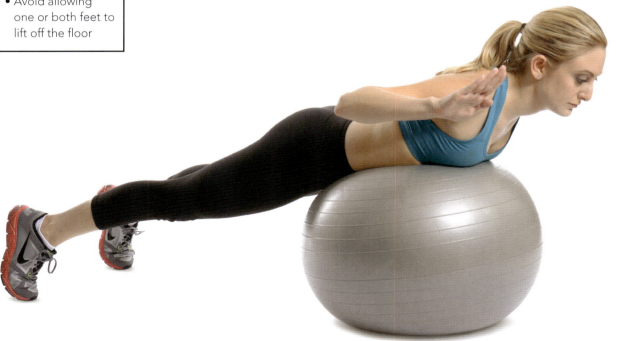

4 Rotate your forearms until they are parallel to the floor.

5 Reverse the movement until your fingers are nearly touching the floor

6 Repeat as prescribed.

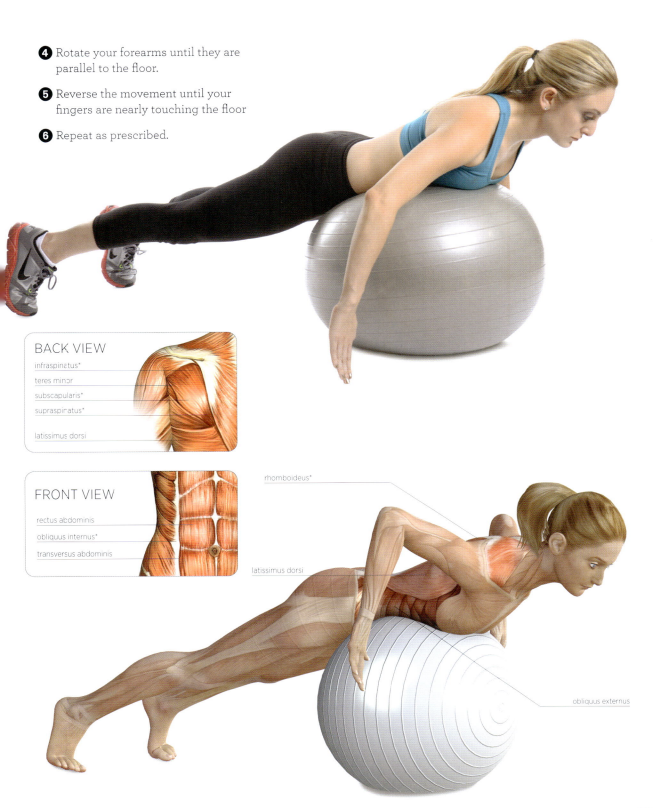

BACK VIEW

infraspinatus*

teres minor

subscapularis*

supraspiratus*

latissimus dorsi

FRONT VIEW

rectus abdominis

obliquus internus*

transversus abdominis

rhomboideus*

latissimus dorsi

obliquus externus

1 MIN TARGETS

BEGINNER
5 x 10-sec reps

INTERMEDIATE
5 x 15-sec reps

ADVANCED
6 x 20-sec reps

BEST FOR

- Quads
- Hamstrings
- Glutes

FIND YOUR FORM

- Keep your feet flexed and your knees pressed together.
- Press equally with both hands.
- Avoid holding your breath
- Avoid twisting your shoulders.

DOUBLE-LEG AB PRESS

Pressing as hard as you can against your quadriceps is a great workout for your core muscles. If this is too difficult, the exercise can be modified by pressing on one leg at a time.

1 Lie on your back with your knees and feet lifted in tabletop position, your thighs making a 90-degree angle with your upper body. Place your hands on the front of your knees, your fingers facing upward, a palm on each leg.

2 Flex your feet and, keeping your elbows bent and pulled into your sides, press your hands into your knees. Create resistance by pushing back against your hands with your knees.

3 Lift your shoulders off the floor. Hold for up to a minute.

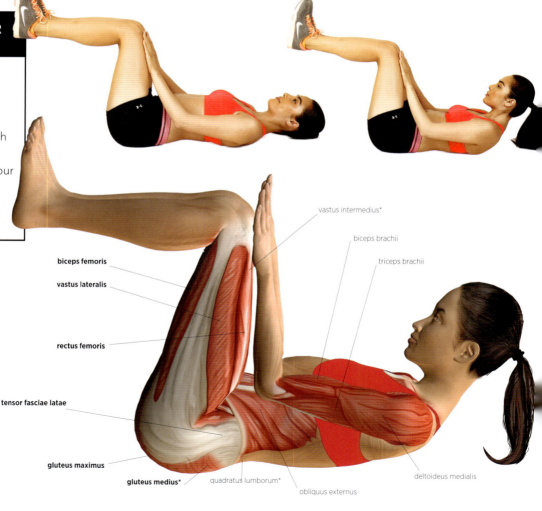

vastus intermedius*

biceps brachii

triceps brachii

biceps femoris

vastus lateralis

rectus femoris

tensor fasciae latae

gluteus maximus

gluteus medius*

quadratus lumborum*

obliquus externus

deltoideus medialis

BEGINNER

15 reps

INTERMEDIATE

20 reps

ADVANCED

40 reps

BEST FOR

- Triceps
- Shoulders
- Abdominals
- Quads

FIND YOUR FORM

- Apply gentle pressure between your elbows and your knees, encouraging your knees to open farther and deepening the inner-thigh stretch.
- Lengthen your spine, keeping your back straight.
- Broaden across your collarbones.
- Avoid rounding your shoulders forward.

CHAIR AB CRUNCH

Chair workouts are great for anyone who spends a lot of time at a desk, and for people with poor balance or limited mobility who can benefit from the support a chair offers. Because your abdominals are a group of smaller, linked muscles, they benefit from daily workouts, and rarely require a day of rest between.

1 Sit on a chair with your hands grasping the sides of the seat and your arms straight.

2 Move your torso forward and if possible lift your buttocks slightly off the chair. Your hips and knees should be bent to form 90-degree angles.

3 In one movement, tuck your tailbone toward the front of the chair and bend your knees toward your chest. As you bend your knees, slightly bend your elbows as well.

4 Keeping your head in a neutral position, extend your elbows and press through your shoulders into the chair and lower your legs to return to the starting position. Repeat as prescribed.

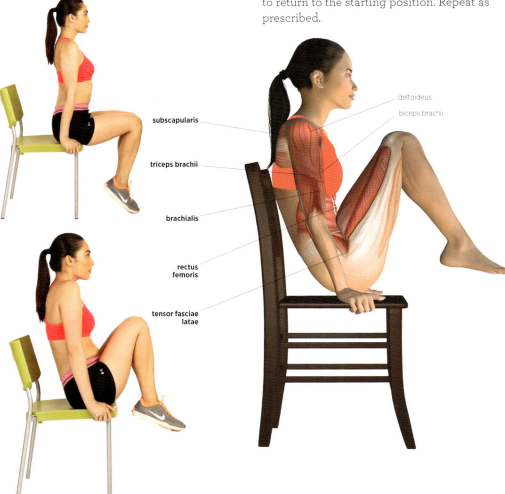

subscapularis

triceps brachii

brachialis

rectus femoris

tensor fasciae latae

deltoideus

biceps brachii

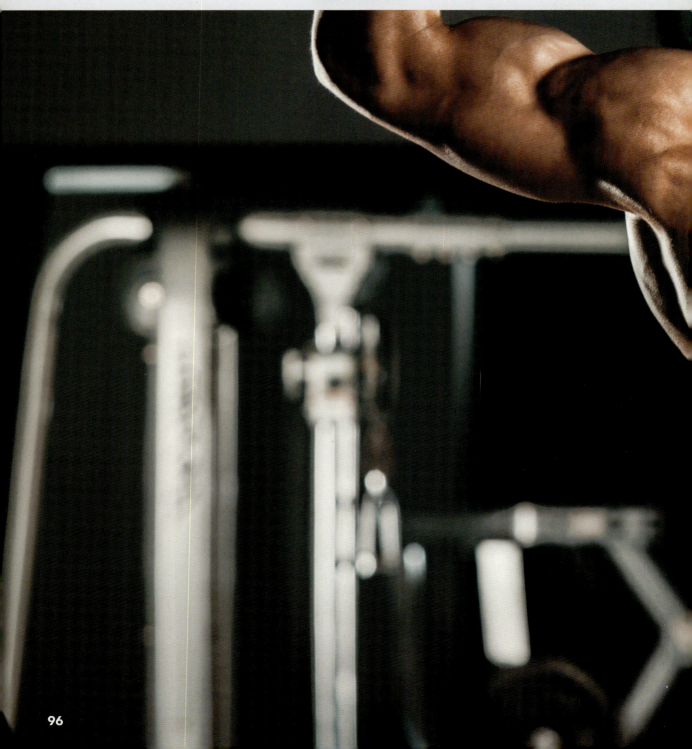

BACK

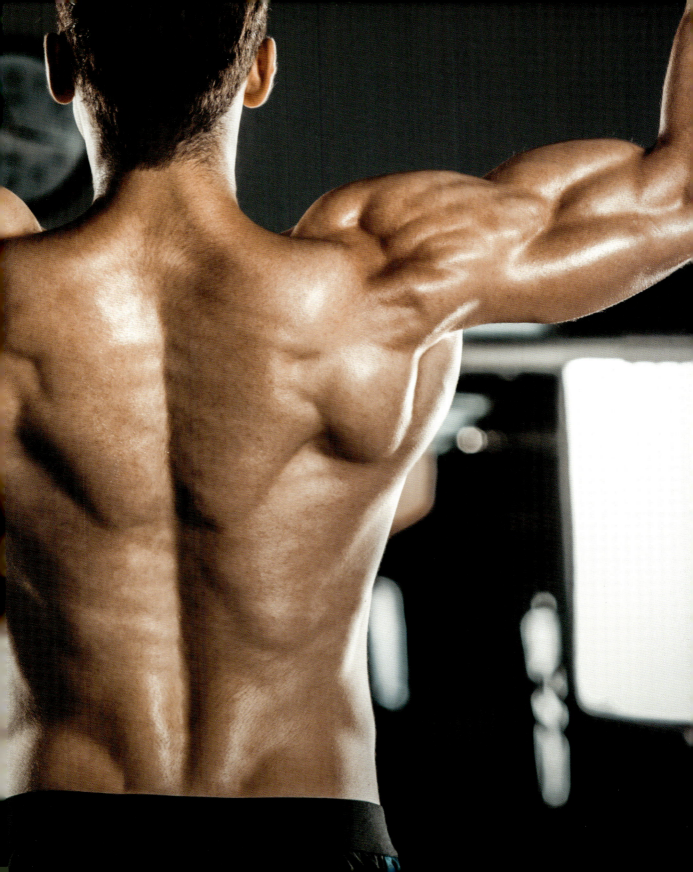

1 MIN TARGETS

BEGINNER
4 x 10 sec holds + rest

INTERMEDIATE
3 x 15 sec holds + rest

ADVANCED
2 x 30 sec holds

BEST FOR

• Spine
• Glutes

FIND YOUR FORM

• Perform a simultaneous movement with your raised arm and leg.

• Keep your hip bones in contact with the floor.

• Avoid any rotation of your torso or hips from the floor.

ARM-LEG EXTENSION

This stretching exercise strengthens your core and back as well as your glutes. The Arm-Leg Extension can also provide relief for a tense lower-back.

❶ Lie flat on the floor. Bend your left arm, and place your palm flat on the floor under your chin.

❷ Extend your right arm, pointing your thumb up toward the ceiling. Simultaneously lift your right arm, torso, and your left leg. Your arm and leg should remain straight as you lift them up to form an arc with your torso.

❸ Slowly lower your arm and leg back down, and then repeat to the opposite side.

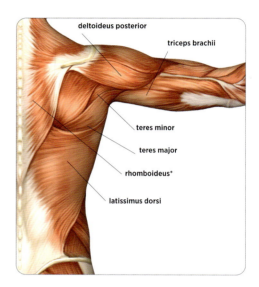

deltoideus posterior
triceps brachii
teres minor
teres major
rhomboideus*
latissimus dorsi

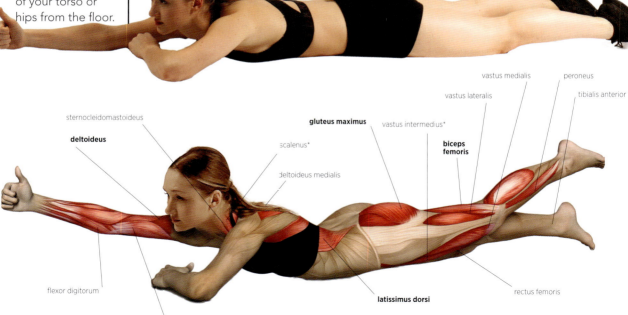

sternocleidomastoideus
deltoideus
gluteus maximus
vastus intermedius*
scalenus*
deltoideus medialis
vastus medialis
peroneus
vastus lateralis
tibialis anterior
biceps femoris
flexor digitorum
rectus femoris
biceps brachii
latissimus dorsi

BEGINNER

4 x 15 sec holds

INTERMEDIATE

4 x 30 sec holds

ADVANCED

6 x 30 sec holds

BEST FOR

• Lower back
• Obliques

FIND YOUR FORM

• Keep your core centered.
• Move carefully and with control.
• Avoid swinging your legs excessively.

HIP CROSSOVER

The Hip Crossover effectively consolidates your core. As with many core exercises, aim for controlled movements. You want your muscles—not momentum—to move you.

1 Lie on your back with your arms lengthened away from your body and your legs bent at a 90-degree angle and lifted off the floor.

2 Brace your abs, and lower your knees to your right side, dropping them as close to the floor as possible without lifting your shoulders off the floor.

3 Return to the starting position, hold for the recommended time, and repeat on the opposite side.

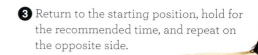

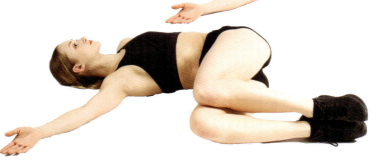

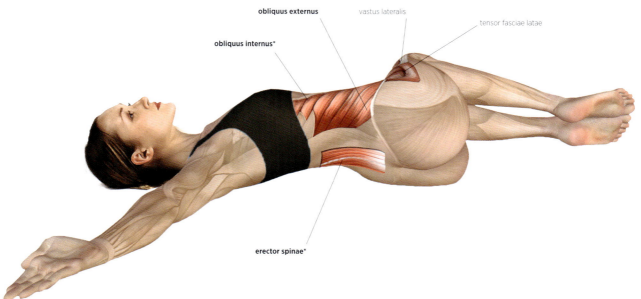

obliquus externus

vastus lateralis

tensor fasciae latae

obliquus internus*

erector spinae*

1 MIN TARGETS

BEGINNER

4 x 10 sec holds + rest

INTERMEDIATE

3 x 15 sec holds + rest

ADVANCED

2 x 30 sec holds

BEST FOR

- Hips
- Spine

FIND YOUR FORM

- Extend your limbs as long as possible in opposite directions.
- Keep your glutes tightly squeezed and your navel drawn in.
- Keep your neck long and relaxed.
- Avoid allowing your shoulders to lift toward your ears.

SWIMMING

An exercise that looks simple, the Swimmer is actually difficult to perform correctly. It engages just about every muscle in your body, but it especially targets your hip extensors, both stretching and strengthening them. It is also an effective back exercise for your back, strengthening the muscles that support your spine.

❶ Lie facedown with your legs hip-width apart. Stretch your arms upward beside your ears on the floor. Engage your pelvic floor, and draw your navel into your spine.

❷ Extend through your upper back as you lift your left arm and right leg simultaneously. Lift your head and shoulders off the floor.

❸ Lower your arm and leg to the starting position, maintaining a stretch in your limbs throughout.

❹ Extend your opposite arm and leg off the floor, lengthening and lifting your head and shoulders.

❺ Elongate your limbs as you return to the starting position. Repeat, alternating sides for the recommended repetitions.

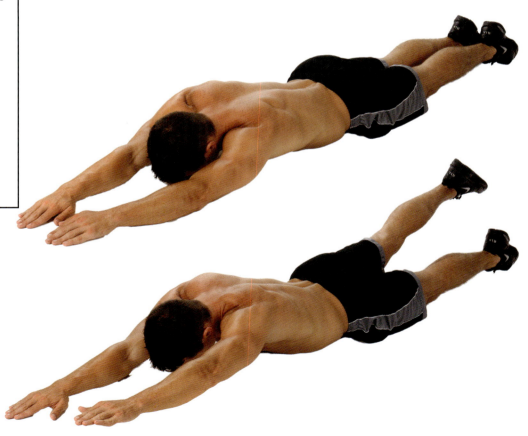

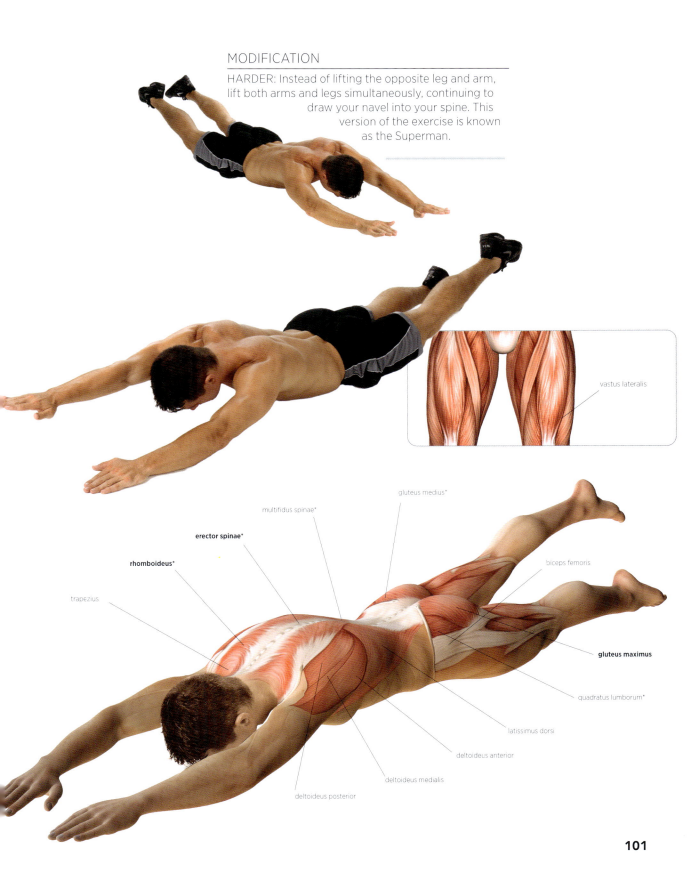

MODIFICATION

HARDER: Instead of lifting the opposite leg and arm, lift both arms and legs simultaneously, continuing to draw your navel into your spine. This version of the exercise is known as the Superman.

vastus lateralis

gluteus medius*

multifidus spinae*

erector spinae*

rhomboideus*

trapezius

biceps femoris

gluteus maximus

quadratus lumborum*

latissimus dorsi

deltoideus anterior

deltoideus medialis

deltoideus posterior

101

1 MIN TARGETS

BEGINNER

4 x 15 sec holds

INTERMEDIATE

4 x 30 sec holds

ADVANCED

6 x 30 sec holds

BEST FOR

- Abdominals
- Back
- Glutes

FIND YOUR FORM

- Move slowly and with control.
- Keep your neck relaxed and your gaze toward the floor.
- Tuck your chin slightly while contracting your arm and leg inward.
- Keep your abs pulled.
- Avoid twisting your torso.
- Avoid arching your back while your arm and leg are extended.

BIRD DOG

The Bird-Dog is an effective exercise for building back, abdominal, and glute strength and developing core body strength. It has the added bonus of improving balance and smooth coordination.

1 Kneel on all fours with your back straight and your abdominals pulled in.

2 Keeping your torso stable and your abdominals engaged, contract your right arm and your left leg into your body.

3 Extend your right arm and left leg outward. Hold the extended position for the recommended time.

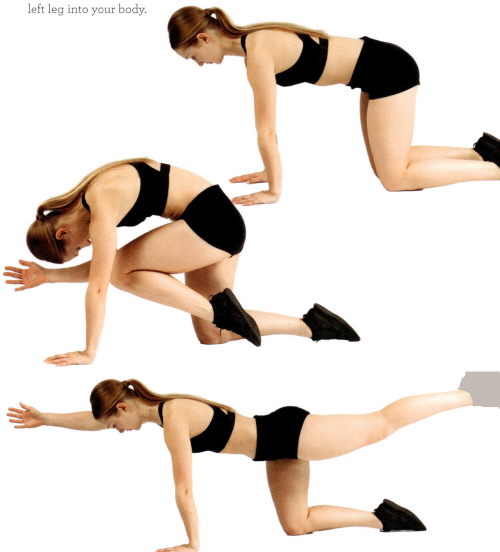

MODIFICATION

HARDER: Instead of kneeling, press into a plank position to begin, and then raise the opposite arm and leg.

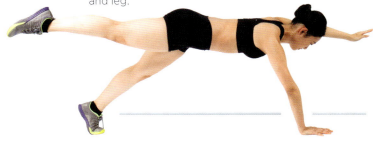

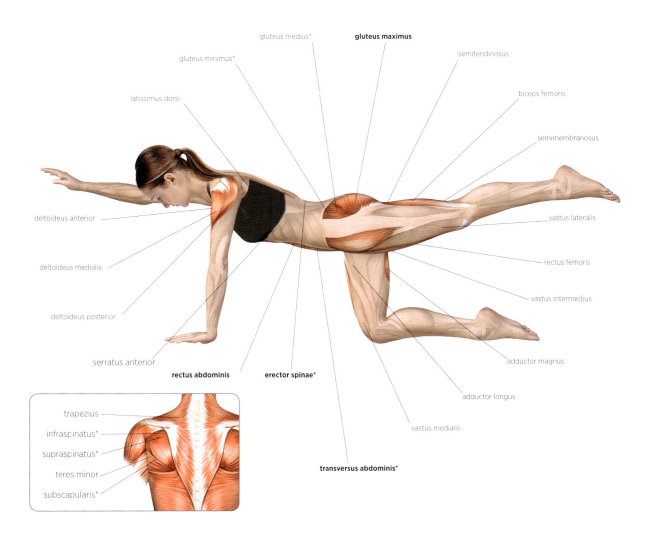

gluteus medius*

gluteus maximus

gluteus minimus*

semitendinosus

latissimus dorsi

biceps femoris

semimembranosus

deltoideus anterior

vastus lateralis

deltoideus medialis

rectus femoris

deltoideus posterior

vastus intermedius

serratus anterior

adductor magnus

rectus abdominis

erector spinae*

adductor longus

vastus medialis

trapezius

infraspinatus*

supraspinatus*

teres minor

subscapularis*

transversus abdominis*

1 MIN TARGETS

BEGINNER

4 x 10 sec holds + rest

INTERMEDIATE

3 x 15 sec holds + rest

ADVANCED

2 x 30 sec holds

BEST FOR

- Lower back
- Abdominals
- Glutes

FIND YOUR FORM

- Complete the full range of motion in both the negative (the downward stretch) and positive (the upward motion) movements of the exercise.
- Avoid overcontracting or hyperextending your back at the top of the movement.

SWISS BALL HYPEREXTENSION

If you do not have access to a gym's hyperextension machine, performing this exercise on a Swiss ball is a great way to work your lower-back muscles. It also strengthens you abdominals and glutes.

1 Lie facedown on top of a Swiss ball, with your abdominals covering most of the ball, your legs spread with toes on the floor, and your arms behind your head. Push your toes into the floor for stability.

2 Raise your torso so that it forms a line with the lower half of your body.

3 Squeeze your glutes as you lower your upper body, and then raise it back to the starting position.

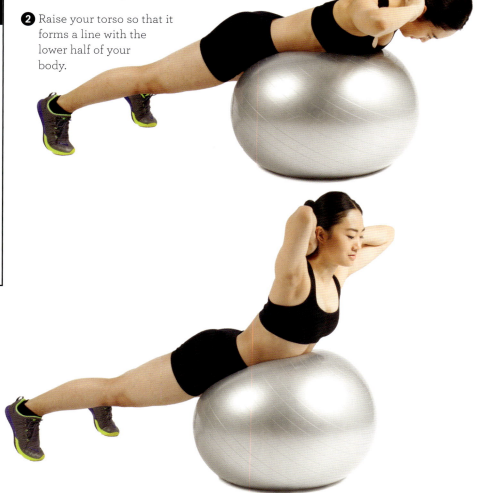

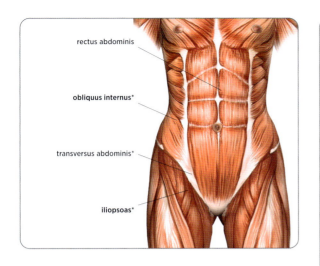

rectus abdominis

obliquus internus*

transversus abdominis*

iliopsoas*

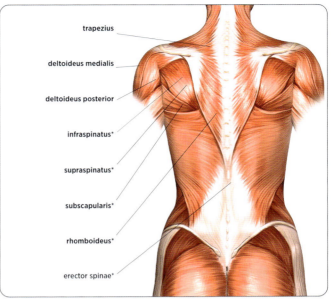

trapezius

deltoideus medialis

deltoideus posterior

infraspinatus*

supraspinatus*

subscapularis*

rhomboideus*

erector spinae*

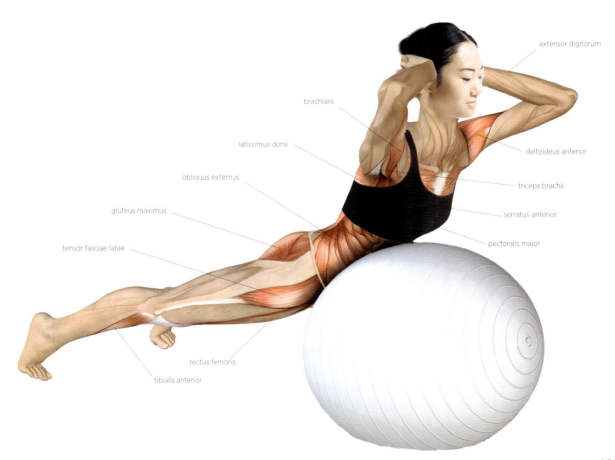

extensor digitorum

brachialis

latissimus dorsi

obliquus externus

gluteus maximus

tensor fasciae latae

deltoideus anterior

triceps brachii

serratus anterior

pectoralis major

rectus femoris

tibialis anterior

1 MIN TARGETS

BEGINNER
4 x 15 sec holds

INTERMEDIATE
4 x 30 sec holds

ADVANCED
6 x 30 sec holds

BEST FOR

- Upper back
- Back extensors
- Obliques

FIND YOUR FORM

- Move carefully—lower yourself to only as far as you feel a distinct stretch. As you become more flexible, you can deepen the stretch.
- Avoid lifting your buttocks off the chair.

CHAIR TWIST

Although this spine-opening movement is simple, perform it carefully: lower your body only until you feel a stretch. As you become more flexible, you can deepen the stretch.

1 Sit upright on a chair, with your legs separated and your feet planted firmly on the floor.

2 Moving slowly, extend your upper back and lean forward while twisting to the left from the waist. Reach your right hand to the front left leg of the chair to stabilize your body.

3 Lift and rotate your torso while keeping your hand firmly on the chair leg.

4 Slowly return to the starting position, and then reach to the right side. Repeat five times in each direction.

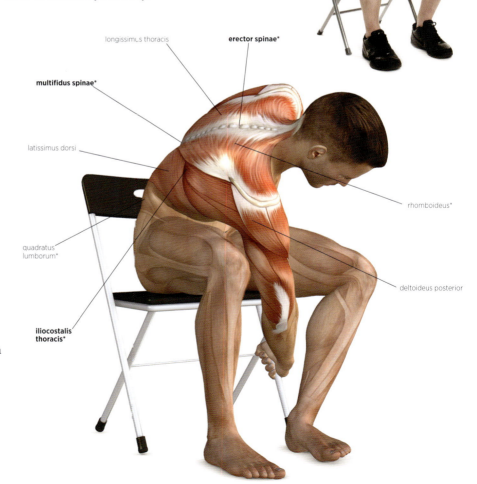

longissimus thoracis

erector spinae*

multifidus spinae*

latissimus dorsi

rhomboideus*

quadratus lumborum*

deltoideus posterior

iliocostalis thoracis*

BEGINNER

20 reps

INTERMEDIATE

30 reps

ADVANCED

40 reps

BEST FOR

• Spine
• Abdominals
• Shoulders

FIND YOUR FORM

• Apply gentle pressure between your elbows and your knees, encouraging your knees to open farther and deepening the inner-thigh stretch.

• Lengthen your spine, keeping your back straight.

• Broaden across your collarbones.

• Avoid rounding your shoulders forward.

BREAST STROKE

The Breaststroke helps to realign your spine, particularly in the upper and middle regions. This exercise strengthens the scapular muscles around the shoulder blades as you rotate your arms, and it develops the extensor muscles as you hold yourself up. If you tend to slouch, this is a great strengthening stretch.

❶ Lie facedown on a mat with your arms and legs extended and your hands shoulder-width apart.

❷ Inhale to prepare, then exhale as you lift your arms off the mat reaching forward.

❸ Slowly circle your arms to the back, so that your fingers are pointed behind you

❹ Bend your elbows, and return to the starting position. Repeat for the recommended repetitions.

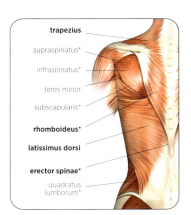

trapezius
supraspinatus*
infraspinatus*
teres minor
subscapularis*
rhomboideus*
latissimus dorsi
erector spinae*
quadratus lumborum*

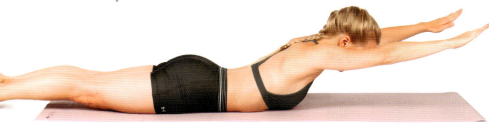

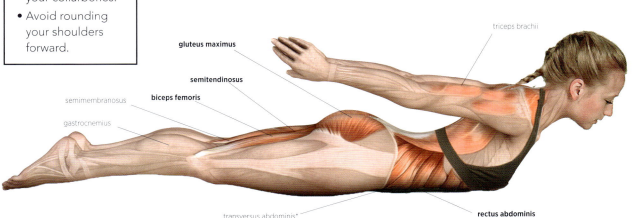

gluteus maximus
semitendinosus
biceps femoris
semimembranosus
gastrocnemius
triceps brachii
transversus abdominis*
rectus abdominis

1 MIN TARGETS

BEGINNER
5 x 10-sec sets

INTERMEDIATE
5 x 15-sec sets

ADVANCED
6 x 20-sec sets

BEST FOR

- Lower back
- Abdominals
- Glutes

FIND YOUR FORM

- Keep your abdominals strong and your hips stable.
- Look toward the floor to elongate your neck.
- Keep your torso and legs still throughout.
- Move your arms from under your shoulder blades.
- Avoid hunching your shoulders.
- Avoid lifting your feet off the floor.

BACK BURNER

The Back Burner strengthens your lower back as well as all of your abdominal muscles. With regular practice, you'll build a strong core while enhancing your posture.

❶ Lie on your stomach with your arms extended in front of you. Your legs should be weighted into the floor with feet pointed. Press your navel to your spine and your shoulders down your back.

❷ Lift your extended arms off the floor and pulse them up and down for the recommended repetitions.

❸ Repeat the movement, this time turning to the left. Return to the center.

❹ Keeping your shoulders down, move your arms to the 3:00 and 9:00 position. Perform a further recommended number of pulses from this position.

❺ Keeping your shoulders down, move your arms to the 3:00 and 9:00 position. Perform a further recommended number of pulses from this position.

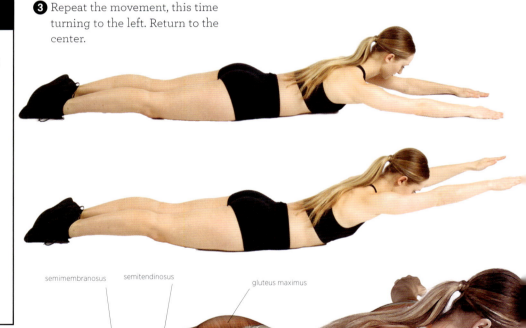

semimembranosus semitendinosus gluteus maximus

biceps femoris

deltoideus posterior

BEGINNER

15 twists each side

INTERMEDIATE

20 twists each side

ADVANCED

30 twists each side

BEST FOR

- Spine
- Shoulders
- Abdominals
- Obliques

FIND YOUR FORM

- Keep your hips facing forward throughout the exercise.
- Avoid raising your hips off the floor.

SPINE TWIST

Stretching and strengthening the back, the Spine Twist is an excellent exercise for increasing the range of motion in the torso and spine, which helps to prevent injury.

1 Sit on the ground with your legs extended and your feet together. Hold your back straight, and raise your arms out to the sides, fully extended, at 90 degrees to your torso.

2 Keeping your abdominals pulled in, twist your waist to the right, taking your entire upper body with it, then return to the central position.

3 Repeat the movement, this time turning to the left. Return to the center.

4 Complete 3 twists in each direction. Stop in the center each time.

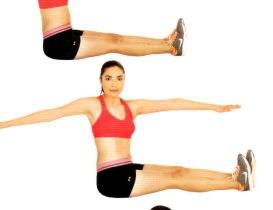

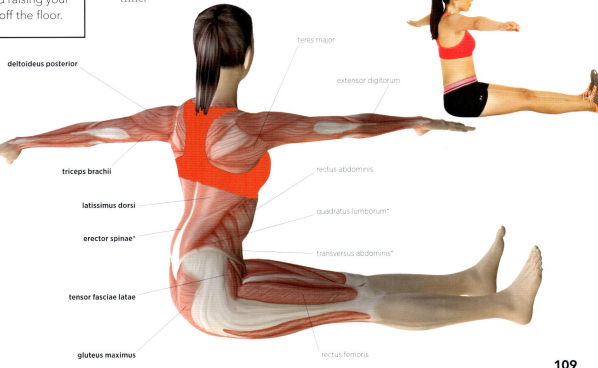

deltoideus posterior

teres major

extensor digitorum

triceps brachii

rectus abdominis

latissimus dorsi

quadratus lumborum*

erector spinae*

transversus abdominis*

tensor fasciae latae

gluteus maximus

rectus femoris

1 MIN TARGETS

BEGINNER

4 x 15 sec holds

INTERMEDIATE

4 x 30 sec holds

ADVANCED

4 x 60 sec holds

BEST FOR

• Rhomboideus

FIND YOUR FORM

• Keep your knees slightly bent.

• Tuck your pelvis forward slightly, allowing your upper body to "contract."

• Imagine a sense of "contraction," as if someone has punched your upper stomach in an upward motion.

• Avoid allowing your knees to turn inward.

STANDING BACK ROLL

The standing Back Roll stretches the Rhomboids—muscles that play a very important part in good posture and a healthy upper back. This is an especially useful exercise if you spend a lot of time working at a desk.

❶ From the bottom position of the Toe Touch, slowly roll up halfway to the point at which you feel your gluteal muscles above your hips and thighs.

❷ Cross your forearms to place your hands on the opposite thighs, and round your shoulders forward.

❸ Feel the heaviness of your head as you stretch your upper back between the shoulder blades.

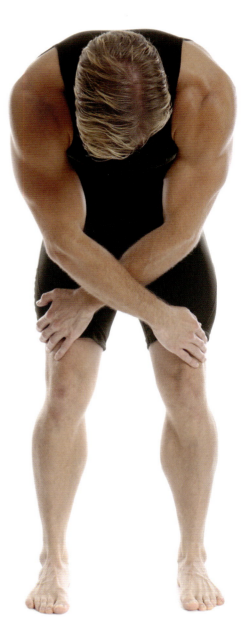

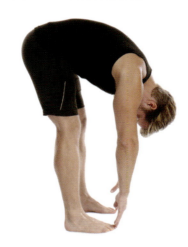

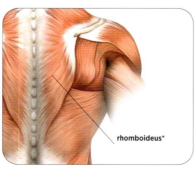

rhomboideus*

BEGINNER

15 bends each side

INTERMEDIATE

20 bends each side

ADVANCED

30 bends each side

BEST FOR

- Back
- Shoulders

FIND YOUR FORM

- Maintain an upright posture.
- Avoid bending forward or backward at the trunk

SIDE BENDS

Side Bends are perfect for stretching the serratus, oblique, and intercostal muscles. This exercise can be modified by placing one hand on your hip and one arm overhead (simpler) or by holding a weight or dumbbell overhead (more difficult). Keep within your comfort zone and increase the stretch over time.

1 Stand with your neck, shoulders, and torso straight.

2 Raise both arms above your head and clasp your hands together, palms facing upward.

3 Leaning from the hips, slowly drop your torso to the left.

4 Keeping a smooth flow, lean your torso to the righ.

5 Slowly repeat the entire sequence 5 times.

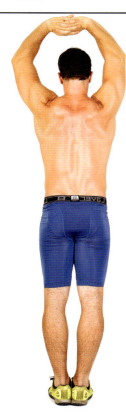

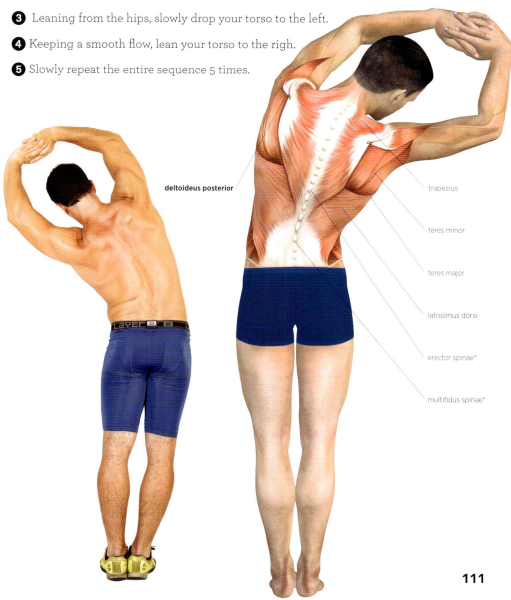

deltoideus posterior

trapezius

teres minor

teres major

latissimus dorsi

erector spinae*

multifidus spinae*

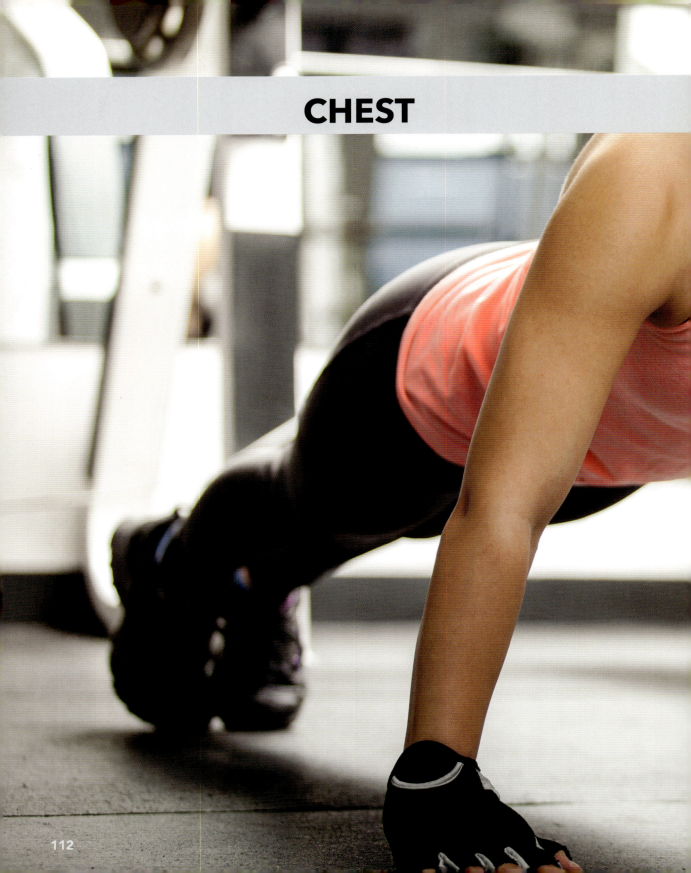

CHEST

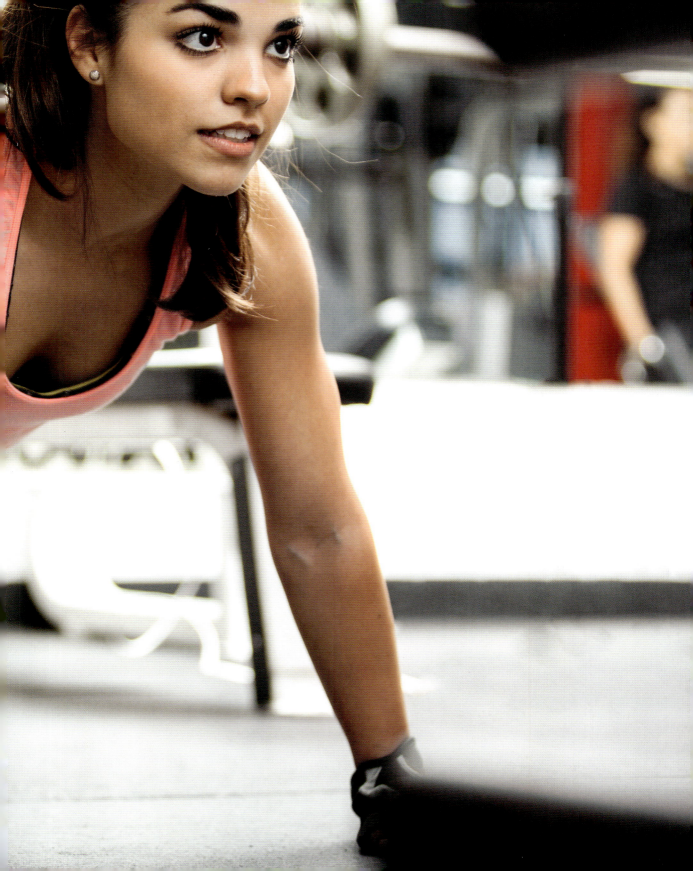

1 MIN TARGETS

BEGINNER
2 sets 8 reps

INTERMEDIATE
2 sets 16 reps

ADVANCED
40 reps

BEST FOR

- Shoulders
- Biceps
- Triceps
- Core

FIND YOUR FORM

- Squat deep, and be sure to keep your thighs parallel to the floor.
- Avoid hyperextending your knees past your toes while squatting.

PUSH-UP

Also known as a press-up, this well-known basic exercise is popular everywhere, from military-style boot camps to Pilates studios. The reason for this is its effectiveness—it really builds power in your core and upper body.

1 Start on your hands and knees, with your hands slightly wider apart than shoulder-width.

2 Push your body up so your arms are straight, with your legs extended backward, to come into a high plank position. Keep your palms on the floor, your feet together, your back straight, and your weight on the balls of your feet. This is your starting position.

3 With control, slowly bend your arms, and lower your torso toward the floor. Lower as far as you can go comfortably—which may be until your chest touches the floor.

4 Straighten your arms to rise back up to your starting plank position. Repeat for the recommended repetitions.

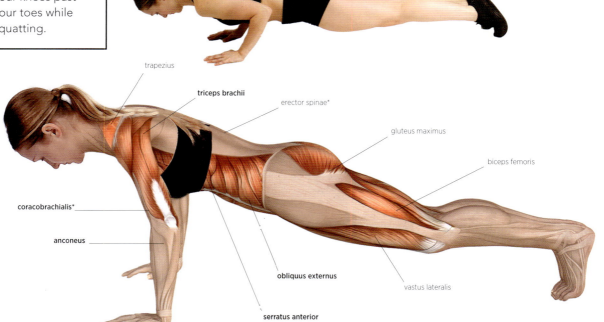

trapezius

triceps brachii

erector spinae*

gluteus maximus

biceps femoris

coracobrachialis*

anconeus

obliquus externus

vastus lateralis

serratus anterior

114

BEGINNER
4 x 15 sec holds

INTERMEDIATE
4 x 30 sec holds

ADVANCED
6 x 30 sec holds

BEST FOR

- Chest
- Ribs
- Hips

FIND YOUR FORM

- Engage your stomach muscles to support your lower back.
- Avoid sinking into your lower back.

THE FISH

The Fish targets your pectoral muscles, the muscles between your ribs, and the iliopsoas muscles of your hips. As with other back-bending yoga poses, the Fish Yoga Stretch is an energizing heart opener that helps to relieve anxiety and fatigue.

1 Lie on your back with your legs flat on the floor. Place your hands beneath your buttocks, and begin to lift your hips off the floor.

2 Press your palms, elbows, and forearms into the floor. Draw your shoulder blades together, and lift your upper back, shoulders, and neck off the floor.

3 Tilt your head back, so the top of your head is touching the floor. Maintain most of your weight on your forearms. Hold for the recommended time, release, and repeat for the recommended repetitions.

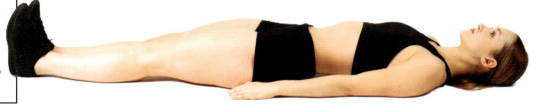

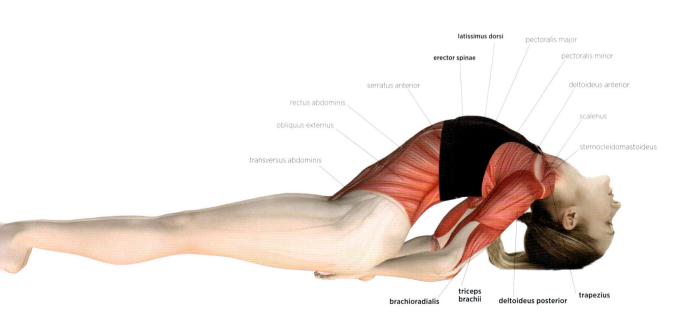

latissimus dorsi

pectoralis major

erector spinae

pectoralis minor

serratus anterior

deltoideus anterior

rectus abdominis

scalenus

obliquus externus

sternocleidomastoideus

transversus abdominis

brachioradialis

triceps brachii

deltoideus posterior

trapezius

1 MIN TARGETS

BEGINNER

2 sets 8 reps

INTERMEDIATE

2 sets 16 reps

ADVANCED

40 reps

BEST FOR

- Triceps
- Biceps
- Shoulders
- Core

FIND YOUR FORM

- Keep your elbows close to your rib cage as you lower your chest toward the floor.
- Keep your spine straight, forming a long line from your tailbone to the crown of your head.
- Avoid pushing your hips into the air.
- Avoid pointing your elbows to the side during the down movement—this places undue stress on the front of your shoulders.

TRICEPS PUSH-UP

Hand position really affects how your muscles are worked—and which ones. In a basic push-up, your pectorals work especially hard. In this version, placing your hands closer together builds strength in your shoulders and triceps.

1 Start on your hands and knees, with your hands fairly close together, about shoulder-width apart, closer than for Push-Up.

2 Push your body up so your arms are straight, with your legs extended backward, to come into a high plank position. Keep your palms on the floor, your feet together, your back straight, and your weight on the balls of your feet. Your wrists should be directly beneath your shoulders, with fingers pointing forward. This is your starting position.

3 With control, slowly bend your arms, and lower your torso toward the floor. Lower as far as you can go comfortably—which may be until your chest touches the floor.

4 Straighten your arms to rise back to the starting position. Repeat for the recommended repetitions.

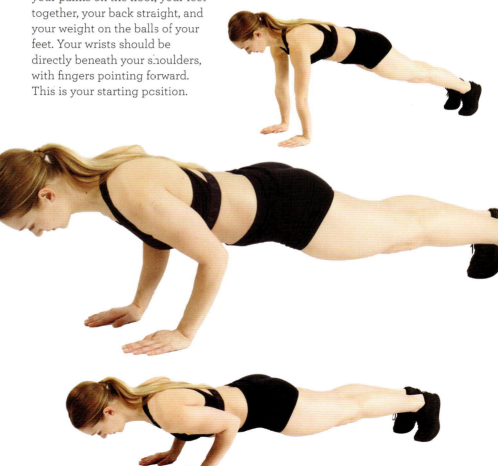

MODIFICATION

EASIER: Start on your hands and knees, with your wrists aligned beneath your shoulders. Lift your feet toward your buttocks until your calves and thighs form a 90-degree angle.

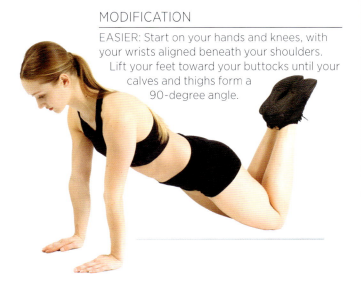

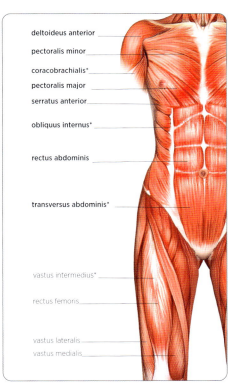

deltoideus anterior
pectoralis minor
coracobrachialis*
pectoralis major
serratus anterior
obliquus internus*
rectus abdominis
transversus abdominis*
vastus intermedius*
rectus femoris
vastus lateralis
vastus medialis

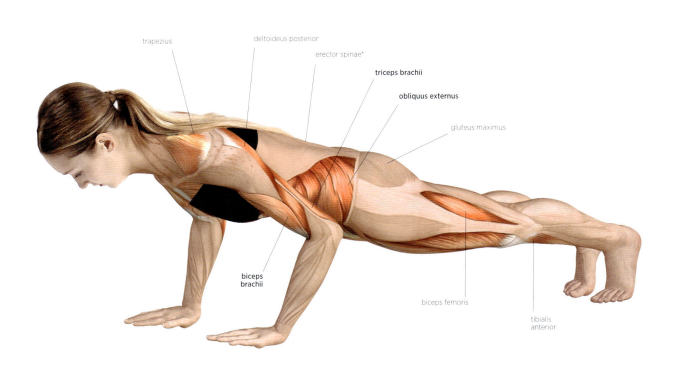

trapezius
deltoideus posterior
erector spinae*
triceps brachii
obliquus externus
gluteus maximus
biceps brachii
biceps femoris
tibialis anterior

1 MIN TARGETS

BEGINNER
4 x 10 sec holds + rest

INTERMEDIATE
3 x 15 sec holds + rest

ADVANCED
2 x 30 sec holds

BEST FOR

• Spine
• Arms
• Legs
• Abdomen

FIND YOUR FORM

• Lengthen your tailbone to create space for your lower back.

• Squeeze your shoulder blades together to help lift your chest.

• Lift your chest and thighs simultaneously.

• Avoid allowing your thighs to rotate outward.

THE BOW

This full backward bend develops spinal strength and flexibility. The Bow is an effective counterpose to forward-bending exercises. It also strengthens your arms, legs, abdomen, and spine.

❶ Lie facedown with your forehead on the floor and your arms at your sides. Press your pelvis and lower abdomen into the floor.

❷ Keep your legs hip-width apart, and bend your knees so that your ankles and shins are in line above your knees.

❸ Inhale, and reach your arms behind you. Grab your ankles, wrapping your hands around the outside of your feet.

❹ Keep your arms straight, as you exhale and lift your chest and thighs from the floor. Pull your feet away from your head to help lift your chest higher.

❺ Rotate your thighs slightly inward. Balance on your navel to find equal extension between the lift of your chest and the lift of your legs.

❻ Hold for the recommended breaths, and release the stretch.

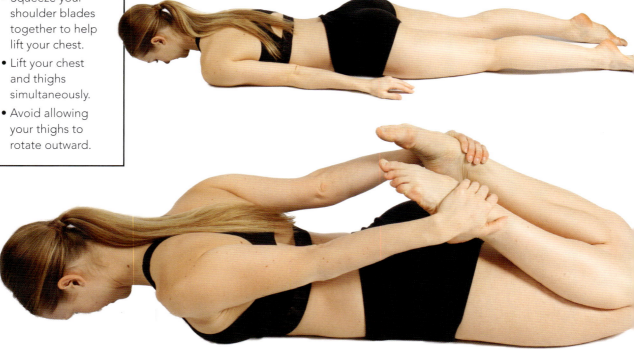

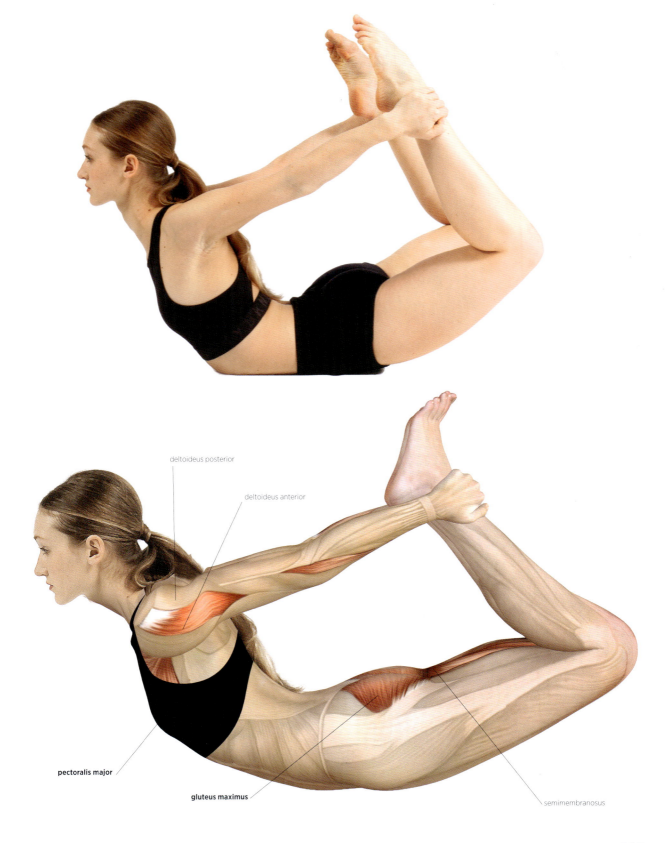

deltoideus posterior

deltoideus anterior

pectoralis major

gluteus maximus

semimembranosus

USH-UP HAND WALK-OVER

The Push-Up Hand Walk-Over adds a dynamic element to the basic push-up. As with any push-up, this variation targets your pectorals and triceps. The added lateral movement also challenges your shoulder and core stabilizers.

❶ Begin in a high plank position, balancing on your toes with your feet together and with your right hand on the floor and your left on an elevated box or step.

❷ Keeping your torso rigid and your legs straight, bend your elbows to lower your chest toward the floor to perform a push-up.

❸ Push back up, straightening your elbows to return to the starting position.

❹ Lift your right hand off the floor, and place it beside your left on the top of the box.

❺ Lift your left hand off the box, placing it on the floor about one shoulder-width to the left, again assuming a high plank position.

❻ Bend your elbows to perform another push-up, this time on the other side of the box.

❼ Return to the top of the box. Continue alternating sides for the recommended repetitions.

ED

r reps

BEST FOR

- Chest
- Shoulders
- Back
- Arms
- Legs

FIND YOUR FORM

- Keep your hands aligned under your shoulders.
- Avoid dipping your shoulders to one side.
- Avoid shifting your hips as your hands walk.
- Avoid craning your neck.

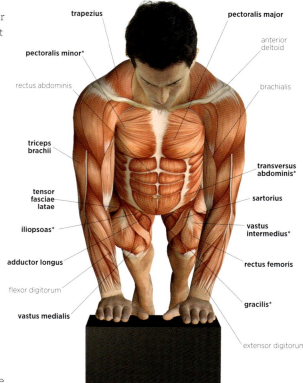

Labels: trapezius, pectoralis major, anterior deltoid, pectoralis minor*, rectus abdominis, brachialis, triceps brachii, transversus abdominis*, tensor fasciae latae, sartorius, iliopsoas*, vastus intermedius*, adductor longus, rectus femoris, flexor digitorum, gracilis*, vastus medialis, extensor digitorum

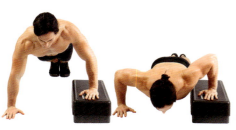
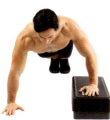
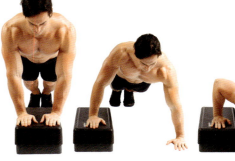

BEGINNER

2 sets 8 reps

INTERMEDIATE

2 sets 16 reps

ADVANCED

40 reps

BEST FOR

• Upper body

FIND YOUR FORM

• Keep your hands planted on the ball.

• Try to keep the ball as still as possible.

• Keep your heels lifted so that you are balancing on your toes.

• Lengthen your spine, keeping your back straight.

• Broaden across your collarbones.

• Avoid rounding your shoulders forward.

BALANCE PUSH-UP

Balance Push-Up is an advanced upper-body exercise. To complete it correctl. demands proper stabilization of your core.

❶ Assume a push-up position with your hands balanced on a fitness ball, shoulder-width apart.

❷ Keeping your body in one straight line, bend your arms and lower your chest until it is nearly touching the fitness ball.

❸ Straighten your arms, pushing to full extension.

❹ Repeat as prescribed.

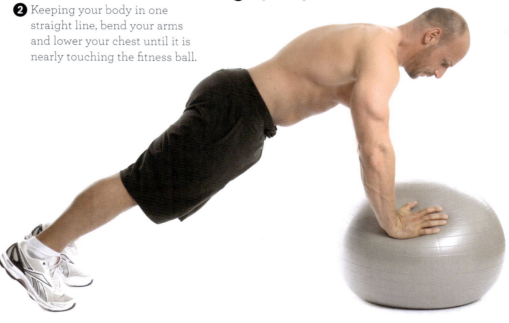

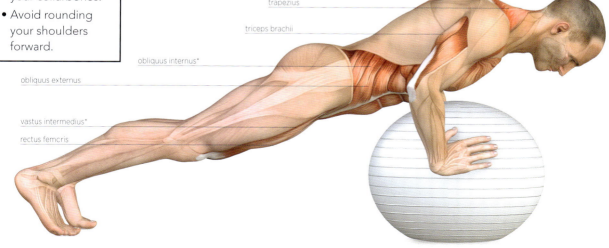

rhomboideus*

trapezius

triceps brachii

obliquus internus*

obliquus externus

vastus intermedius*

rectus femoris

121

WISS BALL WALKAROUND

Swiss Ball Walkaround offers a great challenge for your core stability. It also works your arms and sharpens your sense of balance.

1 Assume a push-up position, with your shins resting on top of the fitness ball.

2 One at a time, "walk" your hands to the side and turn your body so that it rotates in a half circle.

3 Walk your hands in the reverse direction, returning your body to starting position.

4 Repeat, completing the prescribed number of half circles in one direction and then in the other.

.m 10 sets

BEST FOR

- Shoulders
- Abs
- Chest
- Arms

FIND YOUR FORM

- Keep the fitness ball as still and stable as possible.
- Keep your legs, torso, and neck in a straight line.
- Keep your gaze downward.
- Keep your hands' "steps" small enough that you can control the movement.

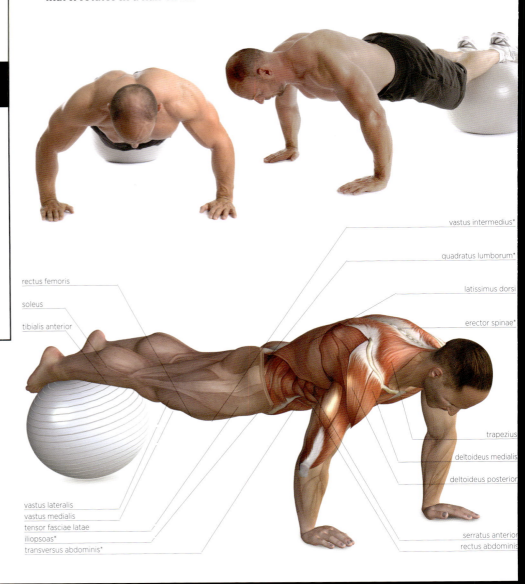

vastus intermedius*

quadratus lumborum*

latissimus dorsi

erector spinae*

rectus femoris

soleus

tibialis anterior

trapezius

deltoideus medialis

deltoideus posterior

vastus lateralis
vastus medialis
tensor fasciae latae
iliopsoas*
transversus abdominis*

serratus anterior
rectus abdominis

BEGINNER

Perform 3 sets of 8

INTERMEDIATE

Perform 5 sets of 8

ADVANCED

Perform 10 sets of 8

BEST FOR

- Chest
- Shoulders
- Abdominals

FIND YOUR FORM

- Apply gentle pressure between your elbows and your knees, encouraging your knees to open farther and deepening the inner-thigh stretch.
- Lengthen your spine, keeping your back straight.
- Broaden across your collarbones.
- Avoid rounding your shoulders forward.

TOWEL FLY

The Towel Fly is an advanced modification of a push-up that calls for you to m
your arms in and out rather than up and down. Utilizing your body weight, it gi
your chest muscles an efficient workout while also recruiting the muscles of you
arms, back, hips, and abdomen to keep your body stabilized. Try to perform as
many as 20 in a row for a high-intensity challenge. You can use a single towel,
two small towels, or even paper plates under your hands—anything that will slide
smoothly on the floor.

1 Place a towel on the floor in front of you. Assume the drop position with your elbows fully extended and a towel under your hands.

2 Maintaining a rigid drop position with your abdominals braced and your weight on your feet, move your hands together. The towel should bunch together below your sternum.

3 Straighten out the towel by pressing outward with your arms, returning to the starting position.

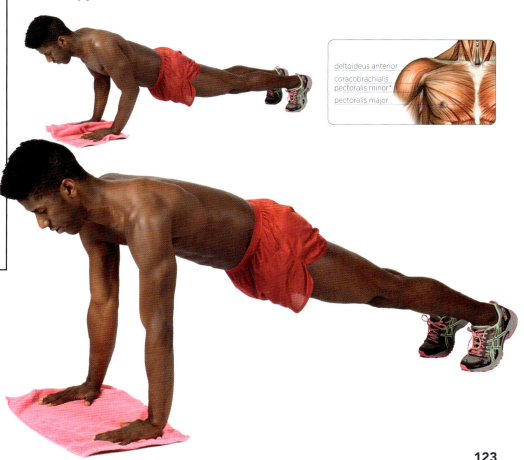

deltoideus anterior
coracobrachialis
pectoralis minor*
pectoralis major

LANK-UP

Plank-Up is an advanced core-stabilizing exercise that expands upon the basic Plank exercise. Try to maintain a steady rhythm as you move from one arm to the other.

❶ Begin on your hands and knees in a facedown position. Plant your forearms on the floor parallel to each other.

❷ Raise your knees off the floor and lengthen your legs until they are in line with your arms.

❸ Raise your knees off the floor and lengthen your legs until they are in line with your arms.

❹ Reverse one arm at a time, lowering from the planted hand to forearm until back in the initial plank position. Repeat as prescribed.

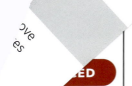

ED

reps

BEST FOR

- Arms
- Core
- Shoulders
- Abs

FIND YOUR FORM

- Plant each hand, rather than using momentum, which places too much stress on the joints.
- Keep your abs tucked tightly during the movement.
- Avoid crashing down suddenly; instead, use a steady 4-count motion: 2 up for both arms, then 2 down.

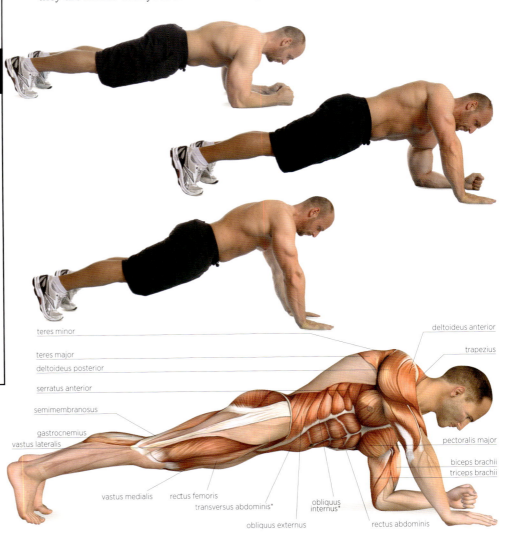

teres minor

teres major

deltoideus posterior

serratus anterior

semimembranosus

gastrocnemius

vastus lateralis

vastus medialis

rectus femoris

transversus abdominis*

obliquus externus

deltoideus anterior

trapezius

pectoralis major

biceps brachii

triceps brachii

obliquus internus*

rectus abdominis

BEGINNER
8 reps

INTERMEDIATE
12 reps

ADVANCED
20 reps

BEST FOR

- Abdominals
- Obliques
- Lower back

FIND YOUR FORM

- Keep your abdominals contracted and tight.
- Keep your body elongated throughout the movement.
- Avoid bridging your back.
- Avoid allowing your hips or lower back to sag.

SWISS BALL ROLLOUT

The Swiss Ball Rollout stabilizes your cores muscles, which prepares them for everyday movements. When performing this exercise, you more effectively act the rectus abdominis and obliques than when performing sit-ups and crunches.

1 Kneel in front of a Swiss ball, and place your hands on it at about hip height.

2 Slowly roll the ball forward, extending your body as you go.

3 While keeping a flat back and remaining anchored on your knees, continue to roll forward until you are completely stretched out.

4 To return to the starting position, engage your abdominal and lower-back muscles and roll back to the starting position. Repeat for the recommended repetitions.

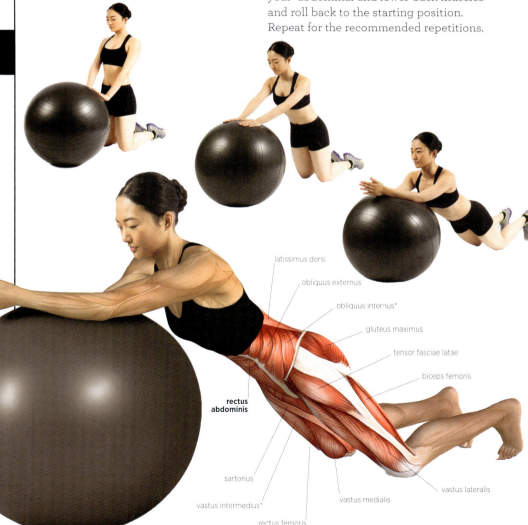

latissimus dorsi

obliquus externus

obliquus internus*

gluteus maximus

tensor fasciae latae

biceps femoris

rectus abdominis

vastus lateralis

vastus medialis

sartorius

vastus intermedius*

rectus femoris

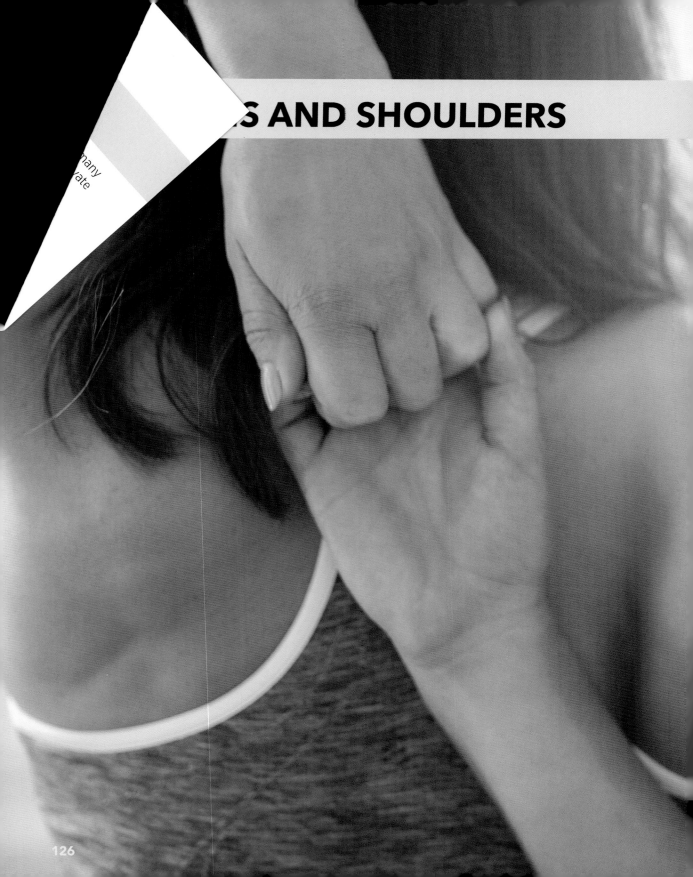

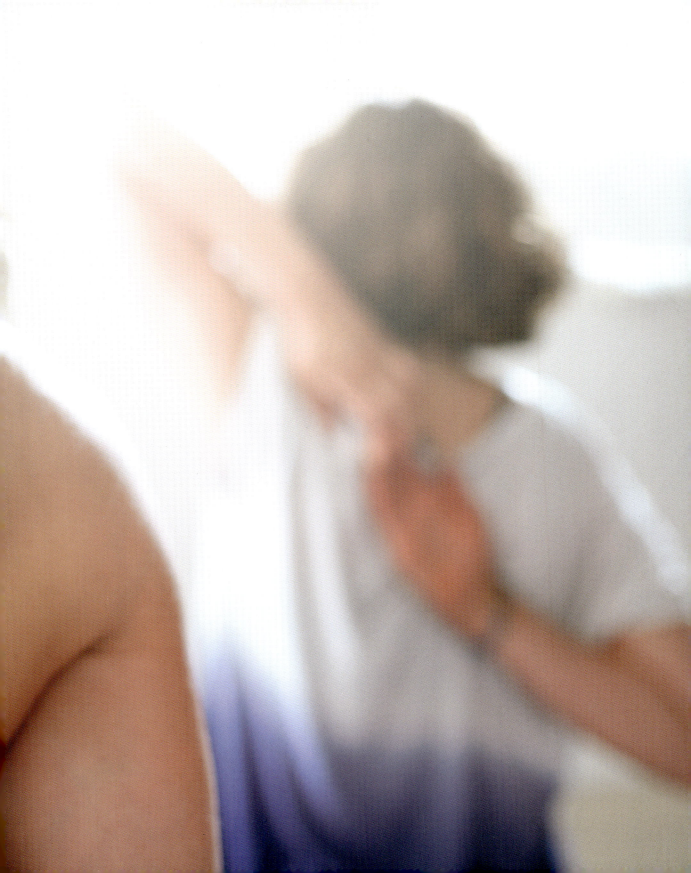

1 MIN TARGETS

BEGINNER

2 sets 8 reps

INTERMEDIATE

2 sets 15 reps

ADVANCED

30 reps

BEST FOR

- Triceps
- Shoulders
- Core

FIND YOUR FORM

- Keep your body close to the chair.
- Keep your spine in a neutral position.
- Avoid allowing your shoulders to lift toward your ears.
- Avoid moving your feet.
- Avoid rounding your back as you lower your hips.
- Avoid pushing up solely with your feet. Instead use your arm strength.

BENCH DIP

The Bench Dip is a classic body-weight exercise that targets your hard-to-isolate triceps. This version replaces a weight bench with an ordinary chair.

1 Sit up tall near the front of a sturdy chair. Place your hands beside your hips, wrapping your fingers over the front edge of the chair.

2 Extend your legs in front of you slightly, and place your feet flat on the floor. Scoot off the edge of the chair until your knees align directly above your feet and your torso will be able to clear the chair as you dip down.

3 Bend your elbows directly behind you without splaying them out to the sides, and lower your torso until your elbows make a 90-degree angle.

4 Press into the chair, raising your body back to the starting position. Repeat for the recommended repetitions.

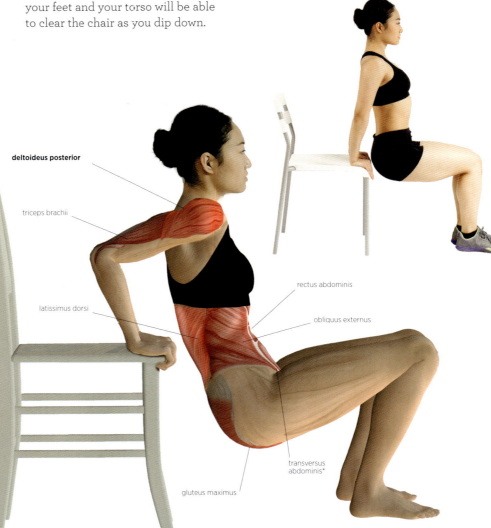

deltoideus posterior

triceps brachii

latissimus dorsi

rectus abdominis

obliquus externus

transversus abdominis*

gluteus maximus

BEGINNER

2 sets 8 reps

INTERMEDIATE

2 sets 15 reps

ADVANCED

30 reps

BEST FOR

- Triceps
- Deltoids
- Pectorals
- Lats

FIND YOUR FORM

- Keep your chest lifted and open.
- Hold your shoulders down.
- Avoid arching your back.
- Avoid lifting your shoulders.
- Avoid rushing through the exercise.

TRICEPS DIP

You should really feel the Triceps Dip on the backs of your arms. Holding this body position works most of your other muscles, too.

1 Sit with your knees bent. Your arms should be behind you with your elbows bent and the palms of your hands pressing into the floor, fingers facing forward. Straighten your arms as you lift your hips a few inches off the floor.

2 Shift your weight back toward your arms, and, keeping your heels pressed firmly into the floor, lift your toes. Keep your chest open and your gaze diagonally upward.

3 Bending your elbows gradually, lower your body down slightly, but still above the floor. Then straighten your arms to raise your body up again, keeping your toes pointed upward the whole time. Repeat the up-and-down action for the recommended repetitions.

4 Release back down to your starting position and repeat for the recommended repetitions.

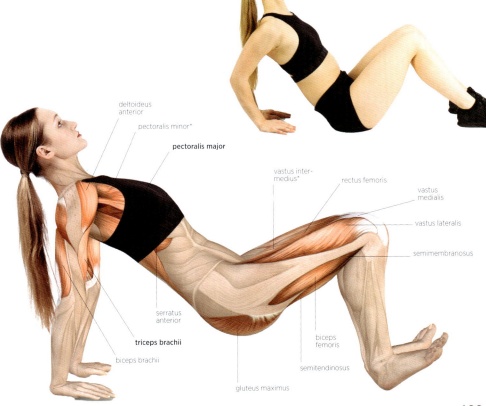

deltoideus anterior

pectoralis minor*

pectoralis major

vastus inter-medius*

rectus femoris

vastus medialis

vastus lateralis

semimembranosus

serratus anterior

triceps brachii

biceps brachii

biceps femoris

semitendinosus

gluteus maximus

1 MIN TARGETS

BEGINNER

2 x 25 sec holds

INTERMEDIATE

2 x 60 sec holds

ADVANCED

Hold 3 mins

BEST FOR

- Quads
- Hamstrings
- Shoulders

FIND YOUR FORM

- Keep your spine straight and abdominals taut. Lengthen your hamstrings and calves. Control the pace of the movement, breathing rhythmically.
- Don't tense your shoulders.

HIGH PLANK PIKE

The Plank Pike is a rejuvenating inversion exercise that improves circulation and reduces neck tension. The Plank Pike lengthens the spine by opening up the space between the individual vertebrae, alleviating spinal compression. And like all planks, it's an excellent full-body workout.

1 Assume a High Plank position with feet hip-width apart.

2 Lift your hips, forming an inverted V-position. Push your heels into the floor and hold for the prescribed time and reps.

3 Pivot your shoulders and hips into High Plank. Hold and repeat as prescribed.

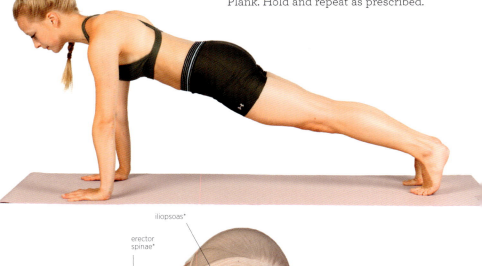

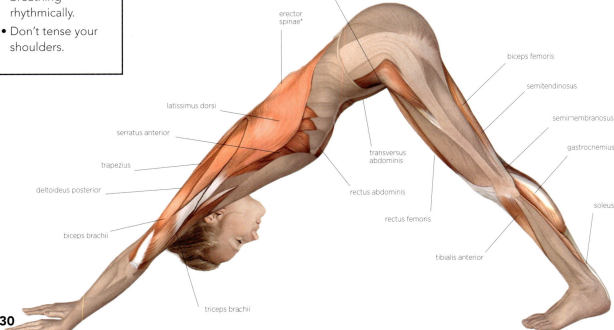

iliopsoas*

erector spinae*

biceps femoris

semitendinosus

semimembranosus

latissimus dorsi

gastrocnemius

serratus anterior

trapezius

transversus abdominis

deltoideus posterior

rectus abdominis

soleus

biceps brachii

rectus femoris

tibialis anterior

triceps brachii

BEGINNER

30 secs each side

INTERMEDIATE

60 secs each side

ADVANCED

2 mins each side

BEST FOR

• Upper body

FIND YOUR FORM

• Keep your fists up and rotate your torso to drive the movement.

• Avoid sloppy form or excessive speed—maintain a steady, even, but modest pace.

POWER PUNCH

You don't have to step into the ring to reap the benefits of boxing, which is a great way to incinerate calories, build strength, and boost stamina. To get the most out of this high-intensity, high-energy kind of workout, you need to get to know the basic fighting stance and punches: the jab, cross, uppercut, and hook. Exercises like the Power Punch lay the groundwork so that you can go on to practice combo moves. You can perform punching exercises alone (in other words, shadowboxing) or you can work with punching bags or a sparring partner.

1 Stand with your feet shoulder-width apart and one leg placed slightly in front of the other, with most of your weight on your back leg. Keep your elbows in and raise your fists up. This is the basic fighting stance.

2 Transferring your weight to your front leg, punch straight in front of you with the fist closest to your body as you turn your torso in to lend power to the punch.

3 Punch for the prescribed time or repetitions, and then reverse sides, switching both arms and legs.

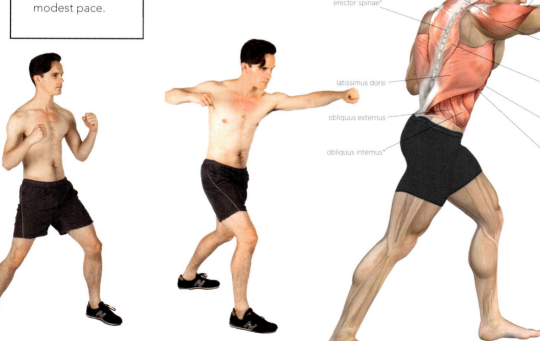

trapezius

deltoideus medialis

erector spinae*

latissimus dorsi

obliquus externus

obliquus internus*

deltoideus anterior

deltoideus posterior

rhomboideus*

serratus anterior

rectus abdominis

BEGINNER

4 r Perform 2 reps eps

INTERMEDIATE

Perform 4 reps

ADVANCED

Perform 8 reps

BEST FOR

- Upper arms
- Back
- Legs
- Glutes

FIND YOUR FORM

- Widen your stance if you have trouble reaching the floor with your hands.
- Keep your abdominals sleek and compact.
- Avoid rushing through the exercise.
- Avoid letting your stomach and spine sag while in the plank position.

INCHWORM

The Inchworm, also known as Monkey Walk, is a full-body stretch that really tests the limits of your flexibility. It is also a good gauge of overall fitness, requiring core and upper-body strength.

1 Stand tall, and then carefully bend forward toward the floor until your palms are flat on the floor in front of you.

2 Slowly walk your hands out to a plank position with your wrists directly under your shoulders. Keep your body parallel to the floor, legs hip-width apart, navel pressing toward your spine and shoulders pressing down your back.

3 Pop your hips upward, and push your weight back onto your heels. Your body should be in the shape of an upside-down V. Hold for a few seconds before slowly walking your hands back toward your legs.

4 Carefully rise back to a standing position. Pause, and then repeat for the recommended repetitions.

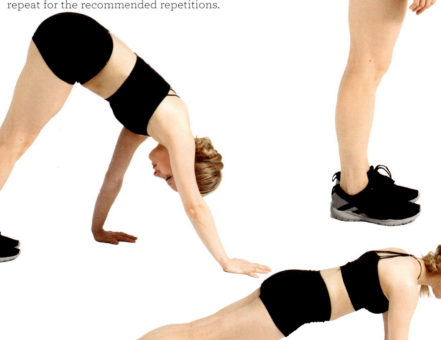

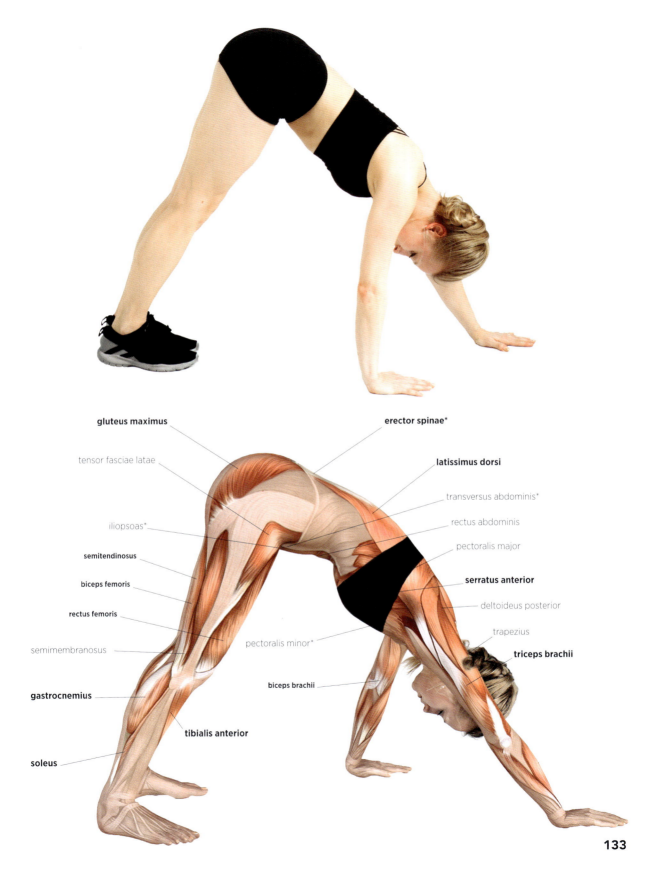

gluteus maximus

erector spinae*

tensor fasciae latae

latissimus dorsi

transversus abdominis*

iliopsoas*

rectus abdominis

semitendinosus

pectoralis major

biceps femoris

serratus anterior

rectus femoris

deltoideus posterior

semimembranosus

trapezius

pectoralis minor*

triceps brachii

gastrocnemius

biceps brachii

tibialis anterior

soleus

133

1 MIN TARGETS

BEGINNER
4 x 5 sec holds

INTERMEDIATE
4 x 10 sec holds

ADVANCED
4 x 20 sec holds

BEST FOR

- Shoulders
- Abdominals
- Legs

FIND YOUR FORM

- Move in a smooth, controlled manner.
- Avoid rolling your shoulders forward—direct them down and apart.

LIFTING UP

This exercise helps prepare you for arm supports and inversions. It not only improves upper-body strength but also engages your abdominals and legs.

1 Begin in Easy Pose. Spread your shoulder blades, and then pull them downward. Practice activating and relaxing your shoulders.

2 Place your hands flat on the floor, fingers facing forward, with elbows straight. Spread your shoulder blades, then pull your shoulders down so that your rib cage lifts up.

3 Press your shoulders down and lift your hips. Lower your hips, and return to a neutral position.

4 Push down with your hands, and lift your hips, leaving your feet on the floor. Lower your hips, and return to a neutral position.

5 To lift your feet, try lifting one knee, then your foot, then your other knee and foot. Lower your hips, and return to a neutral position.

6 Perform the sequence for the recommended repetitions.

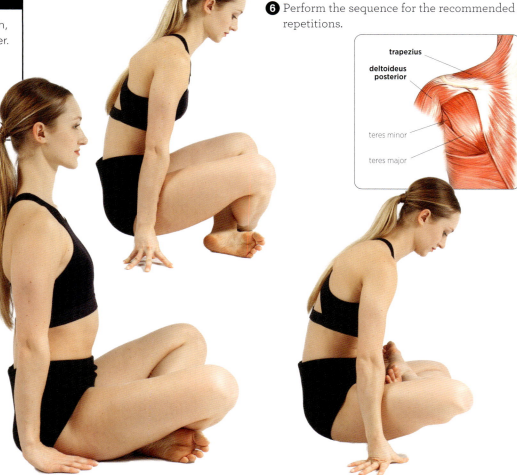

trapezius

deltoideus posterior

teres minor

teres major

1 MIN TARGETS

BEGINNER

2 x 25 sec holds

INTERMEDIATE

2 x 60 sec holds

ADVANCED

Hold 3 mins

BEST FOR

- Core
- Triceps
- Shoulders

FIND YOUR FORM

- Your spine is neutral as you progress through the motion.
- Gaze slightly upward as your lift your body.
- Move smoothly and under control, without force.
- Avoid allowing your shoulders to lift up toward your ears

This is a relatively simple exercise that not only strengthens the triceps and shoulders, but also stretches the back and chest, whilst tightening the muscles in your abs and adductors.

① Lie prone on the floor. Bend your elbows, placing your hands flat on the floor on either side of your chest. Keep your elbows pulled in toward your body. Separate your legs hip-width apart, and extend through your toes. The tops of your feet should be touching the floor.

② Inhale, and press against the floor with your hands and the tops of your feet, lifting your torso and hips off the floor. Contract your thighs, and tuck your tailbone toward your pubis.

③ Lift through the top of your chest, fully extending your arms and creating an arch in your back from your upper torso. Push your shoulders down and back, and elongate your neck as you gaze slightly upward.

④ Hold for the prescribed time, and exhale as you lower yourself to the floor.

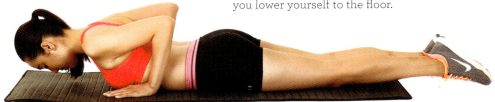

MODIFICATION

EASIER: This exercise can be modified by bending the legs to reduce stress on the abdominals.

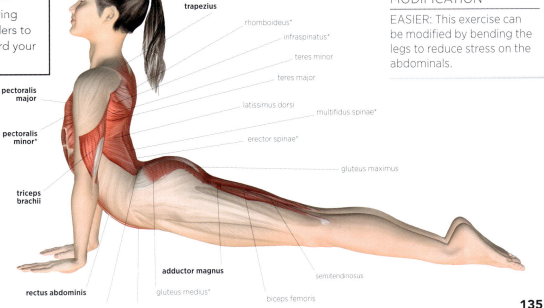

trapezius

rhomboideus*

infraspinatus*

teres minor

teres major

latissimus dorsi

multifidus spinae*

erector spinae*

gluteus maximus

pectoralis major

pectoralis minor*

triceps brachii

rectus abdominis

adductor magnus

gluteus medius*

biceps femoris

semitendinosus

CROW

A graceful asana, Crow Pose strengthens and tones your upper body and serves as an introductory stretch to even more advanced arm balances. Crow Pose is often confused with Crane Pose. The key difference between the two is in your arms: bend your elbows to perform Crow, and keep them straight to perform Crane.

❶ Begin by squatting with your feet and knees more than hip-width apart.

❷ Lean your torso forward, and place your hands in front of you on the mat, facing slightly inward, fingers spread.

❸ Bend your elbows, and rest your knees against your upper arms.

❹ Lifting up on the balls of your feet and leaning forward with your torso, bring your thighs toward your chest and your shins to your upper arms. Round your back as you feel your weight transfer to your wrists. Hold for the recommended recommended amount of time.

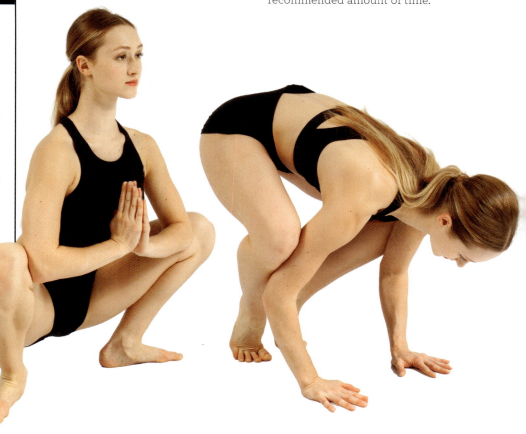

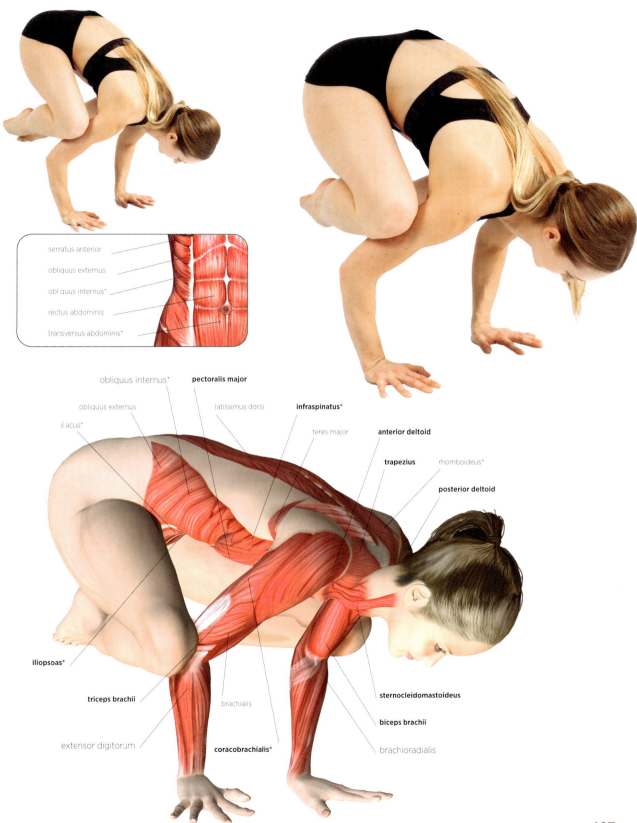

serratus anterior

obliquus externus

obl quus internus*

rectus abdominis

transversus abdominis*

obliquus internus*

obliquus externus

il acus*

pectoralis major

latissimus dorsi

infraspinatus*

teres major

anterior deltoid

trapezius

rhomboideus*

posterior deltoid

iliopsoas*

triceps brachii

brachialis

sternocleidomastoideus

biceps brachii

extensor digitorum

coracobrachialis*

brachioradialis

1 MIN TARGETS

BEGINNER

2 x 25 sec holds

INTERMEDIATE

2 x 60 sec holds

ADVANCED

Hold 3 mins

BEST FOR

- Shoulders
- Arms
- Hamstrings
- Calves

FIND YOUR FORM

- Press your hands fully into the floor at all times to avoid excess strain on your wrist joints.
- Keep your head in line with your spine.
- Keep your back flat and your chest elevated.
- Avoid holding your breath: relax your jaw slightly and breathe normally.

DOWNWARD FACING DOG

Using the strength of your arms and legs to hold your body up, Downward-Facing Dog fully and evenly stretches the length of your spine. It also stretches your hips, hamstrings, and calves while strengthening your quadriceps and ankles. It opens your chest and shoulders and tones your arms and abdominals.

1 Kneel on all fours, with your hands planted directly below your shoulders and your knees aligned beneath your hips.

2 Tuck your toes under, and walk your hands forward about a palm's distance in front of your shoulders. With your hands and toes firmly planted, lift your hips as you straighten your legs and draw your heels toward the floor.

3 Press your chest toward your thighs, and bring your head between your arms. Lengthen through your tailbone, and keep your thighs slightly internally rotated, finding a neutral pelvis. Gaze between your feet or toward your navel. Hold for the recommended time.

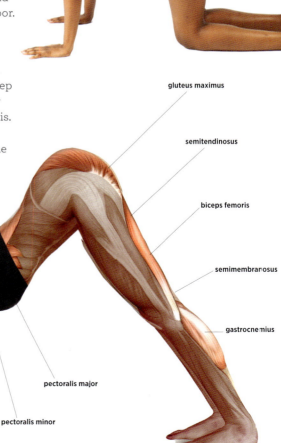

gluteus maximus

semitendinosus

biceps femoris

semimembranosus

gastrocnemius

erector spinae

latissimus dorsi

triceps brachii

pectoralis major

pectoralis minor

1 MIN TARGETS

BEGINNER
4 x 5 sec holds

INTERMEDIATE
4 x 10 sec holds

ADVANCED
4 x 20 sec holds

BEST FOR

- Chest
- Shoulders
- Abdominals
- Hips
- Spine

FIND YOUR FORM

- Elongate the back of your neck.
- Open your chest to extend the arch through your entire spine.
- Avoid bending your knees.

LOCUST

The Locust, a yoga-inspired exercise, involves a mild backbend that stretches your chest, shoulders, and abdominals. It also strengthens your upper and lower back and prepares your body for deeper backbends.

1 Lie facedown on the floor with your arms resting by your sides and the palms of your hands facing downward. Turn your legs in toward each other so that your knees point directly into the floor.

2 Squeezing your buttocks, inhale, and lift up your head, chest, arms, and legs simultaneously. Extend your arms and legs behind you, with your arms parallel to the floor. Lift as high as possible, with your pelvis and lower abdominals stabilizing your body on the floor. Keep your head in a neutral position.

3 Hold for the recommended time, release the stretch, and then repeat for the recommended repetitions.

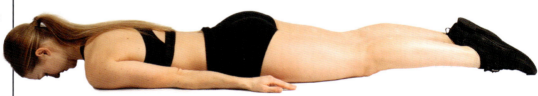

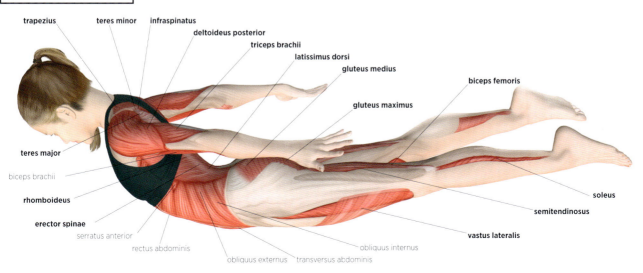

139

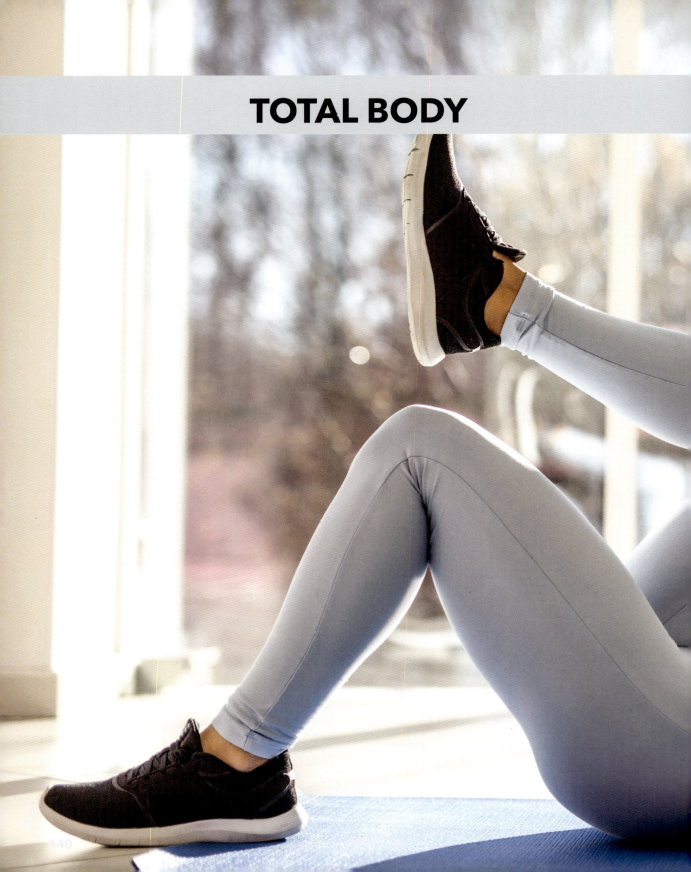

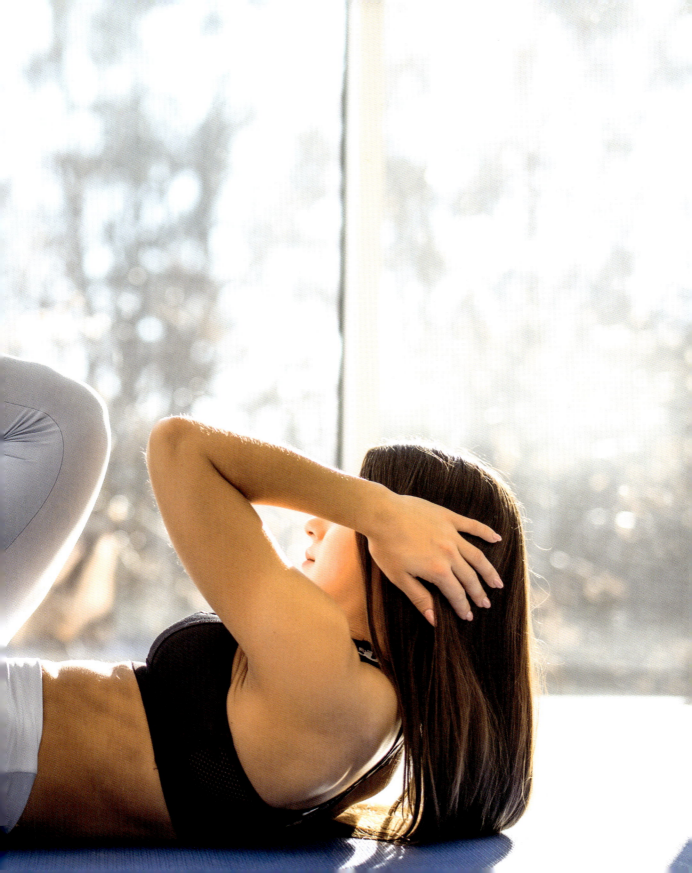

1 MIN TARGETS

BEGINNER
4 sets 10 jumps

INTERMEDIATE
4 sets 15 jumps

ADVANCED
4 sets 25 jumps

BEST FOR

- Shoulders
- Abdominals
- Quadriceps
- Hamstrings
- Glutes

FIND YOUR FORM

- Perform these on a soft surface, such as an exercise mat or padded carpeting, to reduce the impact of your landing.
- Flare out your legs as far as possible.
- Avoid twisting in the jump; landing in an awkward position could cause a torque injury.

STAR JUMP

The Star Jump exercise helps develop leg strength and cardio endurance with the Star Jump. It is not easy as it looks—you must be able to jump high enough to simultaneously extend your legs and arms outward.

1 Stand with your feet together, and then squat down, keeping your knees in line with your toes.

2 In one explosive movement, jump as high as possible while spreading your arms and legs as wide as you can. Your body will make a star shape in the fully extended point of the jump.

3 Bend your knees slightly as you land in the standing position. Sink back to a squat, and repeat. Each jump equals one repetition. Repeat for the recommended repetitions.

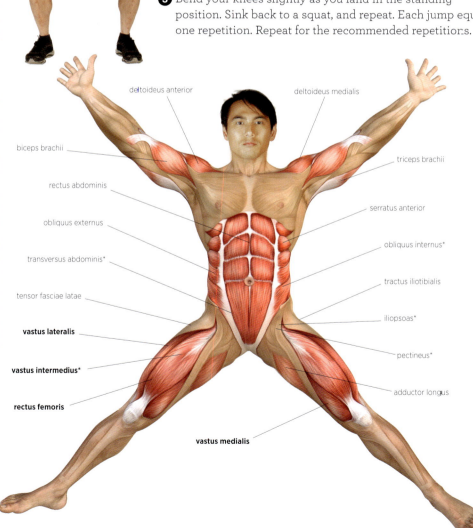

deltoideus anterior

deltoideus medialis

biceps brachii

triceps brachii

rectus abdominis

serratus anterior

obliquus externus

obliquus internus*

transversus abdominis*

tractus iliotibialis

tensor fasciae latae

iliopsoas*

vastus lateralis

pectineus*

vastus intermedius*

adductor longus

rectus femoris

vastus medialis

BEGINNER

Perform for 1 min

INTERMEDIATE

Perform for 2 min

ADVANCED

Perform for 3 min

BEST FOR

- Arms
- Shoulders
- Quads

FIND YOUR FORM

- Move as steadily and as smoothly as possible.
- Avoid placing all of your weight on your arms and shoulders, which can stress your rotator cuffs. Don't let your knees touch the floor.

BEAR CRAWL

The Bear Crawl is a favorite of military special forces around the world, helping to train recruits for real-world movements. Crawling exercises can be tough, but they are great for increasing agility, cardiovascular health, and upper-body strength. They are anaerobic exercises, meaning that they trigger lactic acid formation, which promotes strength, speed, and power.

1 Place both hands and feet on the floor.

2 Walk your left arm and right leg forward, and then your right arm and left leg.

3 Keep moving forward and backward in this position, keeping your weight evenly distributed between your arms and legs.

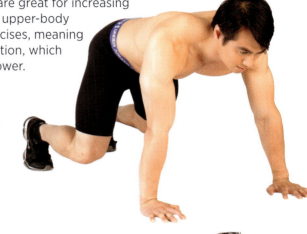

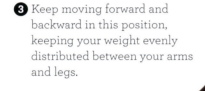

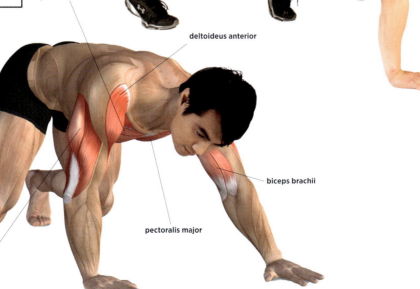

pectoralis minor*

deltoideus anterior

biceps brachii

pectoralis major

triceps brachii

143

1 MIN TARGETS

BEGINNER
Perform for 1 min

INTERMEDIATE
Perform for 2 min

ADVANCED
Perform for 3 min

BEST FOR

- Pectorals
- Deltoids
- Back
- Biceps
- Triceps

FIND YOUR FORM

- Keep your body in a hover position close to the floor, with your elbows at 90 degrees during the entire exercise.
- Avoid allowing your hips to rise.
- Avoid straightening your arms.

ALLIGATOR CRAWL

In the fun but challenging Alligator Crawl, you imitate an alligator stalking its prey. The movements work your chest, shoulders, back, and arms.

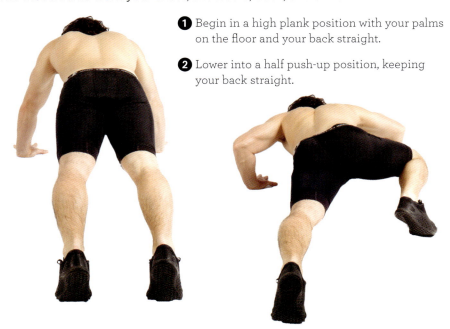

1 Begin in a high plank position with your palms on the floor and your back straight.

2 Lower into a half push-up position, keeping your back straight.

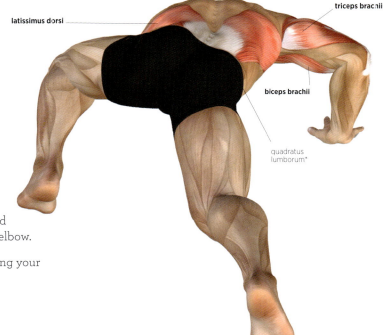

latissimus dorsi

triceps brachii

biceps brachii

quadratus lumborum*

3 Keeping your body low to the floor, bring your right knee to your right elbow while walking your left hand forward.

4 Repeat on the opposite side by walking your right hand forward and bringing your left knee to your left elbow.

5 Continue moving forward, alternating your hand and knee positions. Perform for the recommended time.

LAYOUT PUSH-UP

The Layout Push-Up is an advanced movement requiring intense effort from your back and core musculature. Don't let the "push-up" name fool you because this is not your average gym class exercise—rather than your pectorals, it mainly focuses on your triceps and lats.

1 Lie facedown with your feet together. Stretch your arms upward beside your ears on the floor. Engage your pelvic floor, and draw your navel into your spine.

2 While keeping your core engaged, lift your body up and away from the floor.

3 Lower yourself back to the starting position, and repeat for the recommended repetitions.

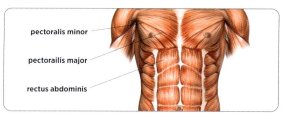

pectoralis minor

pectorailis major

rectus abdominis

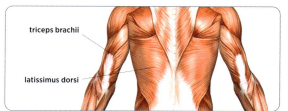

triceps brachii

latissimus dorsi

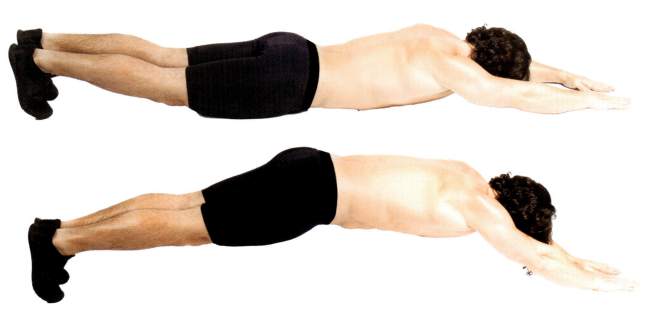

1 MIN TARGETS

BEGINNER

3 reps

INTERMEDIATE

5 reps

ADVANCED

10 reps

BEST FOR

• Total body

FIND YOUR FORM

• Keep your abs engaged throughout the movement.
• Avoid performing the exercise at excessive speed.

TURKISH GET UP

A simple but powerful exercise, the Turkish Get-Up targets multiple muscles throughout your body, including those in the shoulders, core, thighs, back, glutes, and arms. It also increases hip stability and improves balance and coordination.

1 Lie faceup with your legs together. Raise your right arm straight up above your chest and extend your left arm along your side.

2 Flex your right knee, and place your right foot flat on the floor next to your left knee.

3 Rotate your torso slightly to the left, and lift your shoulders off the floor. Plant your left hand on the floor, and lift yourself up to a sitting position.

4 Lift your hips upward, and tuck your left leg under your body to support yourself on your left knee.

5 Lift your left hand off the floor, and push through your right foot to rise to a standing position, keeping your right arm stretched over your head throughout the exercise.

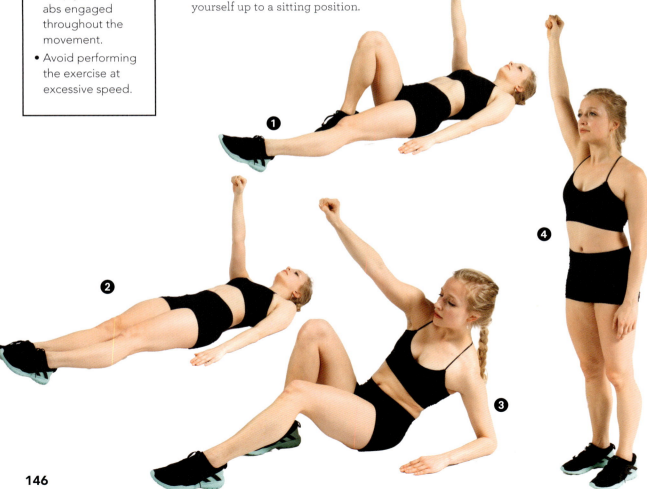

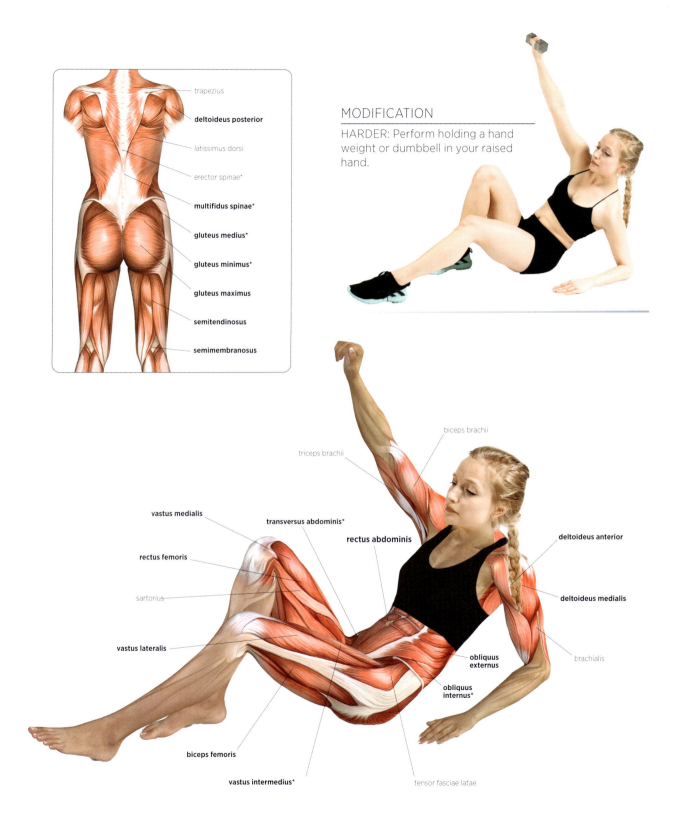

MODIFICATION

HARDER: Perform holding a hand weight or dumbbell in your raised hand.

1 MIN TARGETS

BEGINNER

3 x 15 sec holds

INTERMEDIATE

4 x 20 sec holds

ADVANCED

2 x 2 min holds

BEST FOR

• Total body

FIND YOUR FORM

• Keep your weight evenly distributed along your body. Keep your heels together.

• Keep your weight evenly distributed along your body. Keep your heels together.

PLANK

The Plank offers a full-body workout, strengthening your core, shoulders, arms, legs, and glutes. Because it integrates the whole body, you need to actively coordinate all your mobilization muscles for this exercise. Work up to holding the Plank for 60 seconds.

1 Kneel on all fours, with hands slightly more than shoulder-width apart.

2 Extend your legs behind you in High Plank position, forming a straight line along your back.

3 Pull in your abdominals and hold for a few breaths.

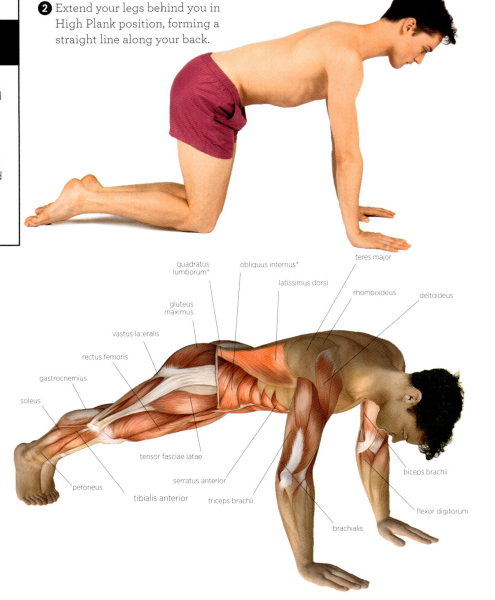

quadratus lumborum*
obliquus internus*
latissimus dorsi
teres major
rhomboideus
deltoideus
gluteus maximus
vastus lateralis
rectus femoris
gastrocnemius
soleus
tensor fasciae latae
serratus anterior
biceps brachii
peroneus
tibialis anterior
triceps brachii
flexor digitorum
brachialis

1 MIN TARGETS	

BEGINNER
3 x 15 sec holds

INTERMEDIATE
4 x 20 sec holds

ADVANCED
2 x 2 min holds

BEST FOR

• Total body

FIND YOUR FORM

• Keep your abdominal muscles tight.
• Keep your body in a straight line.
• Avoid bridging too high, which can take stress off working muscles

FOREARM PLANK

Plank is an isometric, or contracted, core-stabilizing exercise, designed to work your entire core. It is performed everywhere from yoga and Pilates studios to hard-core gyms for a good reason: it is a reliable way to build endurance in your abs and back, as well as in the stabilizer muscles.

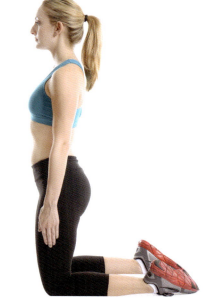

1 Kneel on an exercise mat, and then place your hands on the floor to come into onto all-fours.

2 Plant your forearms on the floor, parallel to each other.

3 Raise your knees off the floor and lengthen your legs until they are in line with your arms. Remain suspended in Plank for 30 seconds, building up to 2 minutes.

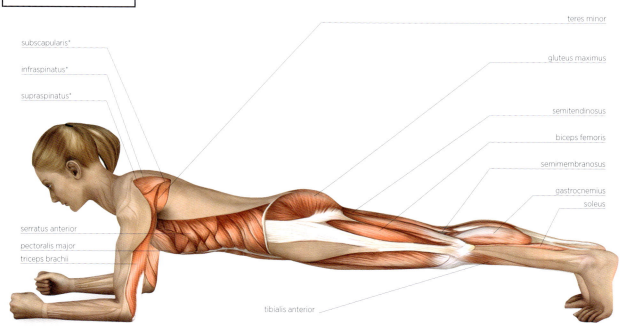

teres minor

gluteus maximus

semitendinosus

biceps femoris

semimembranosus

gastrocnemius

soleus

subscapularis*

infraspinatus*

supraspinatus*

serratus anterior

pectoralis major

triceps brachii

tibialis anterior

1 MIN TARGETS

BEGINNER

3 x 15 sec holds

INTERMEDIATE

4 x 20 sec holds

ADVANCED

2 x 2 min holds

BEST FOR

• Total Body

FIND YOUR FORM

• Contract your abs to have a straight spine.
• Avoid allowing your hips to sink or tilt upward.

ARM-REACH PLANK

Adding an arm-reach tc a plank forces the abs into high gear as they work to keep the torso steady. Balance is key. Place a towel under the elbows if needed.

❶ Begin face-down, resting on your forearms and knees.

❷ One at a time, step your feet back into a plank position. Engage your abdominal muscles and find a neutral spine.

❸ Maintaining proper plank form, slowly lift your right arm off the floor. Hold for prescribed time. Release and return to plank position.

❹ Repeat with the left arm. Aim to increase the hold to prescribed time as you become stronger.

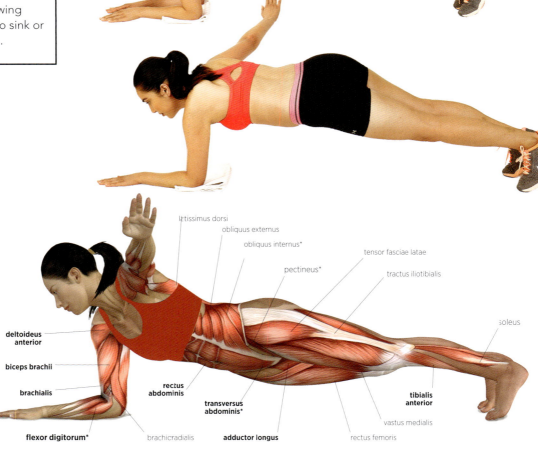

latissimus dorsi
obliquus externus
obliquus internus*
pectineus*
tensor fasciae latae
tractus iliotibialis
soleus
deltoideus anterior
biceps brachii
brachialis
rectus abdominis
transversus abdominis*
tibialis anterior
flexor digitorum*
brachicradialis
adductor longus
vastus medialis
rectus femoris

BEGINNER
3 x 15 sec holds

INTERMEDIATE
4 x 20 sec holds

ADVANCED
2 x 2 min holds

BEST FOR

• Total Body

FIND YOUR FORM

• Elongate your arms and legs as much as possible.

• Keep your feet stacked and flexed.

• Avoid letting your spine or legs fall out of alignment

SIDE PLANK

The challenge of Side Plank Pose lies in maintaining alignment in your spine and legs. Here gravity works against you; try not to let your spine twist, your hips fall forward or lift too high, or your pelvis sink toward the floor. Over time, this will become easier.

1 Begin in Plank Pose with your hands planted on the floor shoulder distance apart, your arms straight and your body lifted off the mat to form a straight line. Your feet should be parallel, with heels lifted. Shift your weight toward the right side of your body, pivoting to the outside edge of your right foot, and stack your left foot on top of your right.

2 On an exhalation, bring your left arm up so that it is perpendicular to the floor. Elongate your body, aiming to form a straight line from head to heels. Turn your head to gaze up toward your left hand.

3 Maintain your balance as you press your right palm into the floor. Hold for prescribed time. Repeat on the other side.

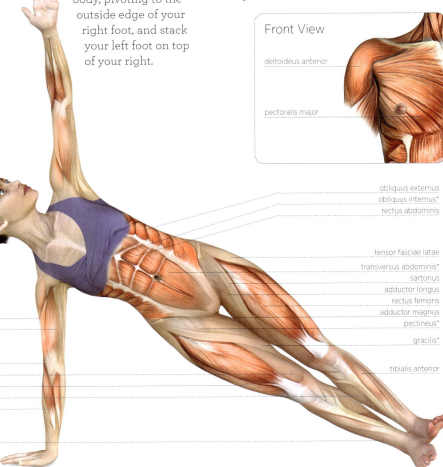

Front View

deltoideus anterior

pectoralis major

obliquus externus
obliquus internus*
rectus abdominis

tensor fasciae latae
transversus abdominis*
sartorius
adductor longus
rectus femoris
adductor magnus
pectineus*
gracilis*

tibialis anterior

brachialis
biceps brachii

brachioradialis
vastus medialis
vastus lateralis
soleus
flexor digitorum*

peroneus

1 MIN TARGETS

BEGINNER

3 x 15 sec holds

INTERMEDIATE

4 x 20 sec holds

ADVANCED

2 x 2 min holds

BEST FOR

• Total body

FIND YOUR FORM

• You should aim to have your entire upper, middle, and lower back flush with the floor underneath you before picking up the body into the elevated position.

• Do not drop the legs so low past the point of being able to keep the abdominals pulling into the body while lying long on the floor.

JACKKNIFE

The Jackknife is a very challenging move that is used in both Pilates and yoga routines. Pulling the legs up overhead from a low extended body position requires abdominal power, balance, and a supple spine. Adding this exercise into your daily workouts will increase core strength and stability throughout the spine, and will help soothe the nervous system by bringing the body upside down.

1 Lie down with your legs extended long out from the hips above you.

2 Scoop the lower abdominals and lower the legs down with your feet pointed.

3 Keeping your back flat along the floor, and the hips still, pull the abs in and lift the legs up, then the hips, then the back, up and over the top of your head. Keep the trajectory of your legs pulling up toward the ceiling.

4 Slowly, control the lowering down of your spine as you return to the starting position.

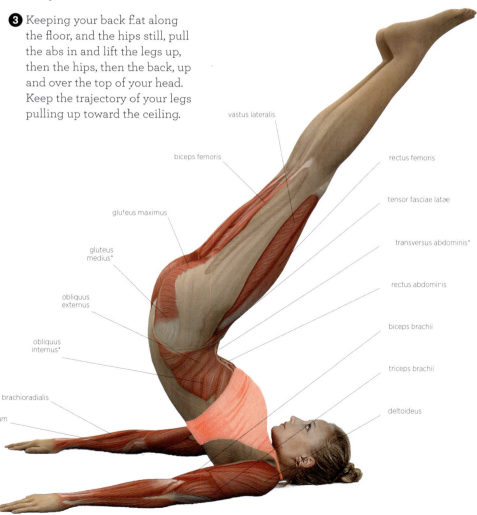

vastus lateralis

biceps femoris

rectus femoris

tensor fasciae latae

gluteus maximus

transversus abdominis*

gluteus medius*

rectus abdominis

obliquus externus

biceps brachii

obliquus internus*

triceps brachii

brachioradialis

deltoideus

extensor digitorum

1 MIN TARGETS

BEGINNER
4 x 10 sec holds

INTERMEDIATE
4 x 20 sec holds

ADVANCED
2 x 2 min holds

BEST FOR

• Total body

FIND YOUR FORM

• Activate your core and gluteal muscles to hold the position. Keep your shoulders above your wrists and lengthen your spine, neck and arms.

• Avoid performing this exercise if you have shoulder or wrist mobility problems.

UPWARD PLANK

The Upward Plank is known by many names—Reverse Plank, Incline Plank, Inclined Plane, and Upward Plane. A basic back-bending yoga pose, it strengthens your core, shoulders, arm, wrist, and leg muscles. It also stretches your shoulders, chest, and ankles while helping you to hone your balance and flexibility.

1 Sit with your legs extended and place the palms of your hands on the floor with fingers facing forward.

2 Move your hands behind your hips, draw your knees toward your chest, and place your feet on the floor with your heels about a foot (30 cm) away from your butt.

3 Press down with your hands and feet and lift your hips until your back and thighs are parallel to the floor with your shoulders directly above your wrists.

4 Without lowering your hips, straighten your legs one at a time. Push your hips higher by lifting your chest and bringing your shoulder blades together, creating a slight arch in your back. Gently elongate your neck and let your head drop back.

5 Hold for the desired time, and then return to the starting position.

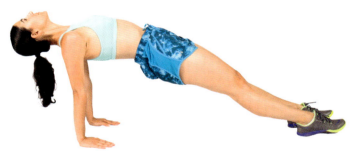

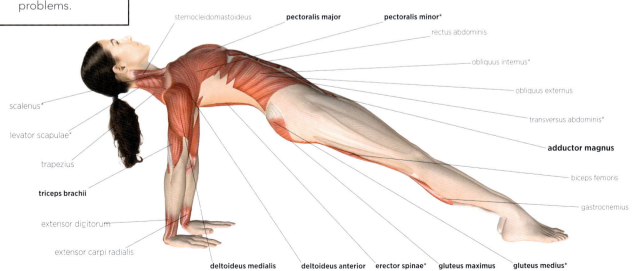

sternocleidomastoideus · **pectoralis major** · **pectoralis minor*** · rectus abdominis · obliquus internus* · obliquus externus · transversus abdominis* · **adductor magnus** · biceps femoris · gastrocnemius

scalenus* · levator scapulae* · trapezius · **triceps brachii** · extensor digitorum · extensor carpi radialis · **deltoideus medialis** · **deltoideus anterior** · **erector spinae*** · **gluteus maximus** · **gluteus medius***

1 MIN TARGETS

BEGINNER

3 x 15 sec holds

INTERMEDIATE

4 x 20 sec holds

ADVANCED

2 x 2 min holds

BEST FOR

• Total body

FIND YOUR FORM

• Keep the back of your neck long by gazing slightly beyond the edge of your mat.

• Avoid bending your elbows so much that your chest collapses and your shoulders round forward.

• Avoid dropping your hips lower than your shoulders.

CHATURANGA PLANK

Chaturanga, sometimes called Four-Limbed Staff Pose, challenges your core strength and stability. It is also an effective strengthener for the arms, legs, and shoulders.

1 Begin in Plank Pose with your hands planted on the floor shoulder distance apart, your arms straight and your body lifted off the mat to form a straight line. Your feet should be parallel, with heels lifted. Exhale as you bend your elbows over your wrists and lower yourself down so that your shoulders are in line with your elbows. As you lower, ground your palm and fingers down into the floor. The thumb and index finger have a tendency to want to lift up, so make a special effort to press down between the two.

2 Hold the pose, rotating your inner thighs and drawing your tailbone downward so that you don't sink into your lower back. Lift your thighs away from the floor. Draw your shoulder blades together as you lift the heads of the shoulders away from the floor.

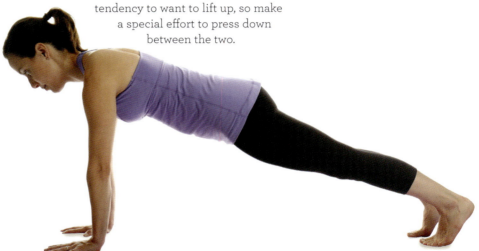

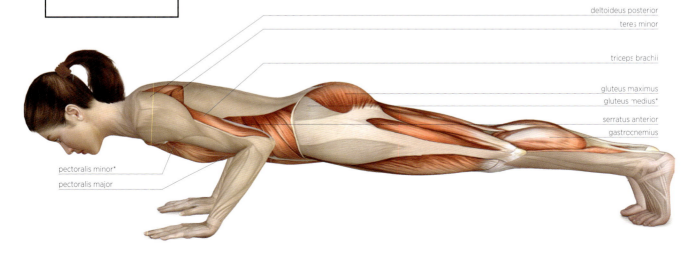

deltoideus posterior

teres minor

triceps brachii

gluteus maximus

gluteus medius*

serratus anterior

gastrocnemius

pectoralis minor*

pectoralis major

BEGINNER

3 x 15 sec holds

INTERMEDIATE

4 x 20 sec holds

ADVANCED

2 x 2 min holds

BEST FOR

• Total body

FIND YOUR FORM

• To challenge yourself, prop as little of your legs on the ball as possible.

• Don't allow your middle back to sag.

SWISS BALL SHIN PLANK

This version of a plank on a Swiss ball is slightly easier than a forearm version. The Swiss Ball Shin Plank is still an effective exercise, helping to stabilize and strengthen your core, back, shoulders, and chest muscles. It also forms the foundation of many other plank moves, preparing you for higher intensity exercises.

❶ Kneel on your hands and knees with a Swiss ball behind you. Raise your legs to rest your shins and ankles on the ball.

❷ Push the ball back to lift and straighten your knees until your body forms a straight line from shoulders to feet.

❸ Hold this position for as long as possible.

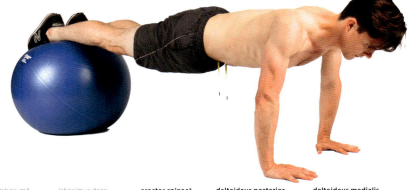

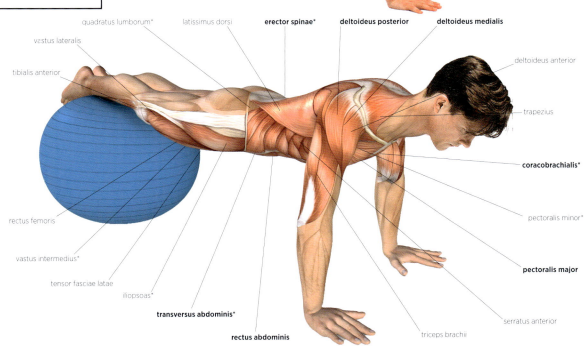

quadratus lumborum*

latissimus dorsi

erector spinae*

deltoideus posterior

deltoideus medialis

vastus lateralis

tibialis anterior

deltoideus anterior

trapezius

coracobrachialis*

rectus femoris

pectoralis minor*

vastus intermedius*

tensor fasciae latae

iliopsoas*

transversus abdominis*

rectus abdominis

pectoralis major

serratus anterior

triceps brachii

WHEEL

The invigorating and energizing Wheel Pose is a deep, challenging backbend that strengthens the entire body, and stretches the chest and rib cage. It is excellent for the heart, liver, and kidneys, and can be beneficial to those who suffer from asthma and osteoporosis.

1 Begin by lying on your back, with your knees bent and your feet hip-width apart. Inhale and stretch your arms straight up to the ceiling, with your palms facing away from you. Then, bend your arms and place your hands on the floor next to your ears, shoulder-width apart, with your fingers facing the same direction as your toes.

2 Press your hands and feet into the floor as you lift your hips up, as if you were coming into Bridge Pose.

3 Lift yourself onto the crown of your head. Pause and press your palms into the floor, spreading your fingers wide and grounding down through every knuckle and through the base of your thumb and index finger.

4 Straighten your arms, and move your outer upper arms inward to find external rotation. Press down through all four corners of your feet, shifting your weight onto your heels. Roll your inner thighs toward the floor as you firm your outer hips inward. Let your head fall between your shoulders in a comfortable position. Hold for the recommended breaths.

5 To come out of the pose, bend your arms and shift your body weight toward your shoulders as you slowly descend, landing on the back of your head and your shoulder blades.

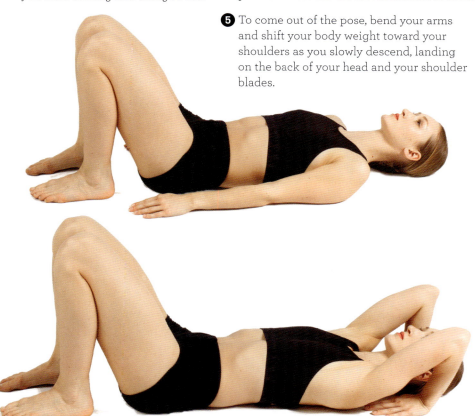

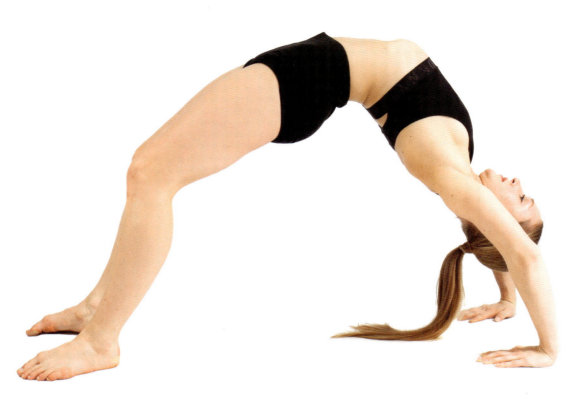

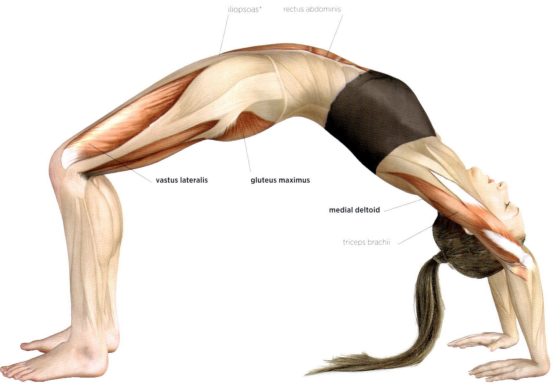

iliopsoas*   rectus abdominis

vastus lateralis   gluteus maximus

medial deltoid

triceps brachii

157

1 MIN TARGETS

BEGINNER

3 x 15 sec holds

INTERMEDIATE

4 x 20 sec holds

ADVANCED

2 x 2 min holds

BEST FOR

• Total body

FIND YOUR FORM

• Keep your abdominal muscles tight and your body in a straight line.

• Your neck should be in a neutral position, not extended or crunched.

• Avoid letting your hips or buttocks sink too low or rise too high.

DOLPHIN PLANK WITH REACH

This more challenging variation of Plank Pose is effective in strengthening your forearms, upper arms, shoulders, and back. It also improves your stamina and posture by building up the muscles that support your spine. Swimmers, gymnasts, and dancers can all benefit from this pose.

1 Begin on all fours with your toes curled forward and facing the front of your mat.

2 Plant your forearms on the floor parallel to each other. Raise your knees off the mat and lengthen your legs until they are in line with your arms. Your body should form a straight line from your shoulders to your heels.

3 Maintaining proper plank form, slowly raise your right arm off the mat and extend it away from your shoulder, fingers outstretched.

4 Hold for the recommended breaths, release the pose, and then repeat on the opposite side.

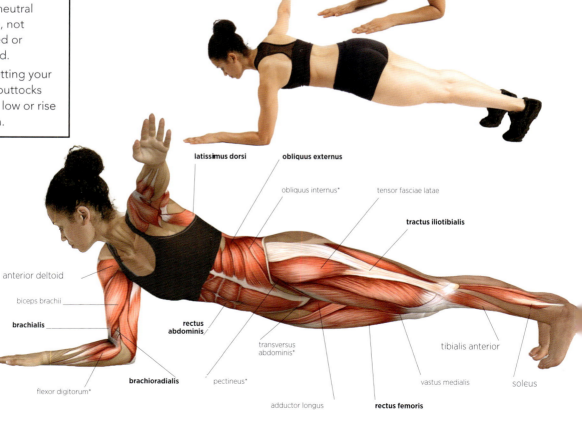

latissimus dorsi

obliquus externus

obliquus internus*

tensor fasciae latae

tractus iliotibialis

anterior deltoid

biceps brachii

brachialis

rectus abdominis

transversus abdominis*

tibialis anterior

brachioradialis

pectineus*

vastus medialis

soleus

flexor digitorum*

adductor longus

rectus femoris

BEGINNER

3 x 15 sec holds

INTERMEDIATE

4 x 20 sec holds

ADVANCED

2 x 2 min holds

BEST FOR

• Total body

FIND YOUR FORM

• Keep your body in one straight line.
• Avoid arching or bridging your back.

T-STABILIZATION

T-Stabilization, another advanced variation on the traditional Plank, is a proven exercise for targeting your abs, hips, lower back, and obliques.

1 Assume the finished push-up position with your arms extended to full lockout, your fingers facing forward, your legs outstretched, and your body weight supported on your toes.

2 Turn your hips to one side, stacking one foot on top of the other and raising your top arm across your body until you are pointing toward the ceiling.

3 Hold for 30 seconds, lower, and then repeat on the other side. Work your way up to holding for prescribed time.

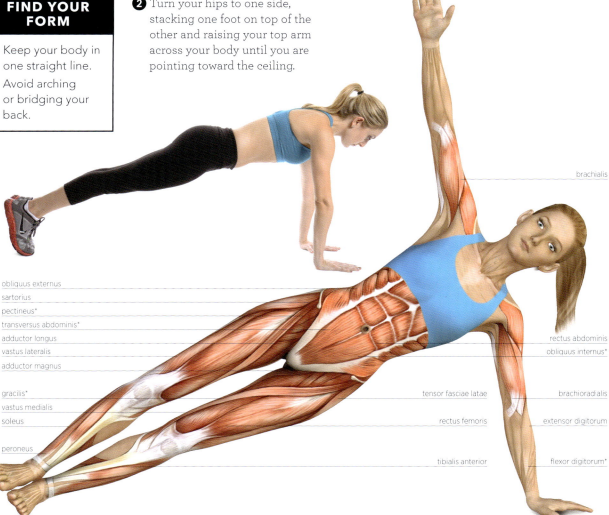

brachialis

obliquus externus

sartorius

pectineus*

transversus abdominis*

adductor longus

vastus lateralis

adductor magnus

gracilis*

vastus medialis

soleus

peroneus

rectus abdominis

obliquus internus*

tensor fasciae latae

brachioradialis

rectus femoris

extensor digitorum

tibialis anterior

flexor digitorum*

1 MIN TARGETS

BEGINNER

4 x 10 sec holds

INTERMEDIATE

4 x 20 sec holds

ADVANCED

2 x 2 min holds

BEST FOR

• Total body

FIND YOUR FORM

• If you're having difficulty rolling over, bend your knees slightly or place a rolled-up towel under your hips.

• Avoid using momentum to push through the movement.

ROLLOVER

Borrowed from Pilates, the Rollover requires a strong core and a controlled, fluid progression. With time and practice, you can perfect this spinal stretch and core strengthener by engaging your abs, articulating your spine, and breathing deeply.

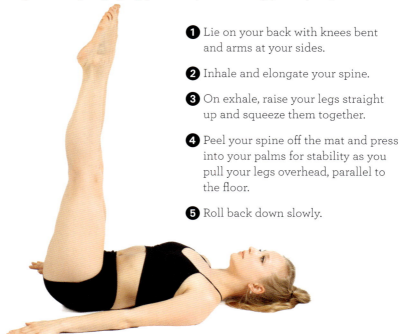

❶ Lie on your back with knees bent and arms at your sides.

❷ Inhale and elongate your spine.

❸ On exhale, raise your legs straight up and squeeze them together.

❹ Peel your spine off the mat and press into your palms for stability as you pull your legs overhead, parallel to the floor.

❺ Roll back down slowly.

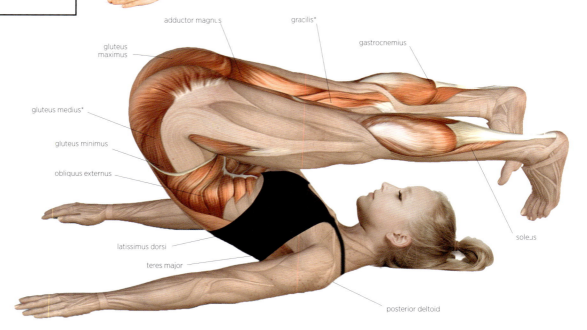

adductor magnus

gracilis*

gastrocnemius

gluteus maximus

gluteus medius*

gluteus minimus

obliquus externus

soleus

latissimus dorsi

teres major

posterior deltoid

SUPERMAN

Superman engages just about every muscle in your body, but it is especially effective at stretching and strengthening the hip flexors. It is also an effective exercise for your back, strengthening both the full extent of the erector spinae, as well as the multifidus spinae. Beware though—this move is harder than it looks.

❶ Lie facedown on your stomach with your arms and legs extended on the floor.

❷ Raise your arms and your legs simultaneously, squeezing your glutes at the top.

❸ Lower, and then repeat.

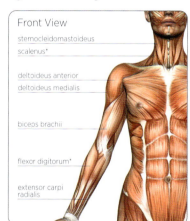

Front View

sternocleidomastoideus
scalenus*
deltoideus anterior
deltoideus medialis
biceps brachii
flexor digitorum*
extensor carpi radialis

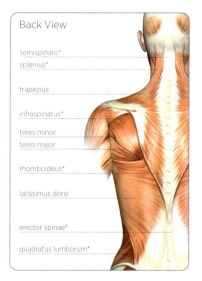

Back View

semispinalis*
splenius*
trapezius
infraspinatus*
teres minor
teres major
rhomboideus*
latissimus dorsi
erector spinae*
quadratus lumborum*

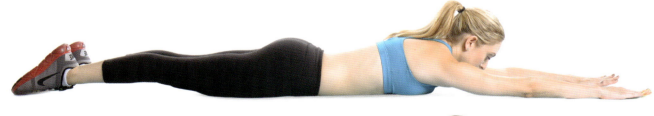

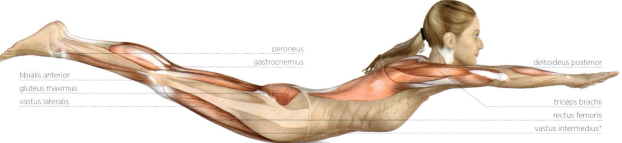

peroneus
gastrocnemius
tibialis anterior
gluteus maximus
vastus lateralis
deltoideus posterior
triceps brachii
rectus femoris
vastus intermedius*

1 MIN TARGETS

BEGINNER
3 x 15 sec holds

INTERMEDIATE
4 x 20 sec holds

ADVANCED
2 x 2 min holds

BEST FOR

• Total body

FIND YOUR FORM

• Try to keep your hips stable and aligned throughout the exercise. Keep a straight line from your shoulders to your knees.
• Don't drop your hips or pelvis as you raise and lower your legs.

TABLETOP MARCH

Building on the basic Bridge the Tabletop March requires you to hold the Bridge position while incorporating leg lifts and lowers.

1 Lie on your back with knees bent and arms at your sides.

2 Exhale and curl your back off the mat, one vertebra at a time. Inhale and lift your left leg into tabletop position, flexing your foot. Lower your foot.

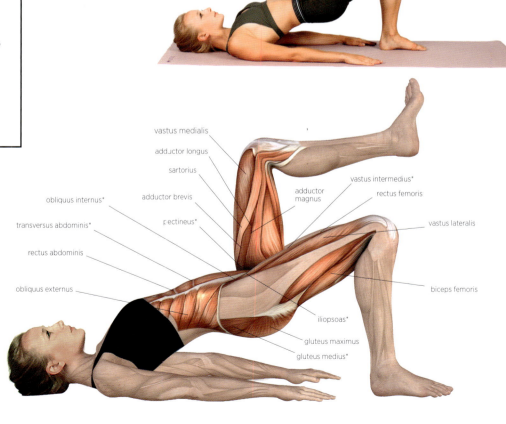

vastus medialis
adductor longus
sartorius
obliquus internus*
adductor brevis
transversus abdominis*
pectineus*
rectus abdominis
obliquus externus
vastus intermedius*
adductor magnus
rectus femoris
vastus lateralis
biceps femoris
iliopsoas*
gluteus maximus
gluteus medius*

BEGINNER

2 sets 8 reps

INTERMEDIATE

2 sets 15 reps

ADVANCED

30 reps

BEST FOR

- Total body

FIND YOUR FORM

- Make sure all movement happens at the same time.
- Keep your shoulders relaxed throughout.
- Avoid allowing your shoulders to lift toward your ears.
- Avoid allowing your hips and lower back to drop during the movement.
- Avoid arching your back.

FOAM ROLLER TRICEPS ROLLOUT

As its name suggests, this exercise is great for your triceps. However, it's also a winning routine for core strength—achieved by engaging the abdominals, pecs, and glutes.

1 Kneel on the floor, with the foam roller placed crosswise in front of you. Place your hands on top of the roller, your fingers pointing away from you.

2 Maintaining a neutral spine and making sure not to sink your into your shoulders, roll forward on your forearms.

3 Continue to roll forward until the roller reaches your elbows. Press into the roller, keeping your hips aligned, and roll back to the starting position. Repeat for the recommended repetitions.

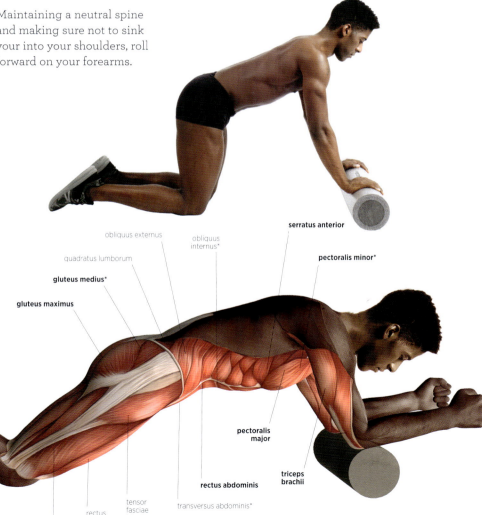

serratus anterior

obliquus externus

obliquus internus*

pectoralis minor*

quadratus lumborum

gluteus medius*

gluteus maximus

pectoralis major

triceps brachii

rectus abdominis

transversus abdominis*

vastus lateralis

rectus femoris

tensor fasciae latae*

1 MIN TARGETS

BEGINNER

4 reps

INTERMEDIATE

8 reps

ADVANCED

15 reps

BEST FOR

• Total body

FIND YOUR FORM

• You must strongly engage the abdominals and core throughout the Burpee movement. It is the only way to move through it smoothly.

• Do not let the lower back sink down while in your plank movement.

• Keep your alignment tight and secure.

BURPEE

The Burpee is said to be one of the best exercises in the world! It is not an easy move to perform, but if you can master it the results are astounding. Performing Burpees correctly can benefit you in many areas: aerobic endurance, dynamic explosive power, core strength, and cardiovascular health.

❶ With feet apart and under your hips, raise the arms up to the sky.

❷ In one move crouch down, placing your hands to floor.

❸ Explode out into a plank position. Then quickly return to the crouched position.

❹ Last, fling your arms up to the air, leaping high with energy.

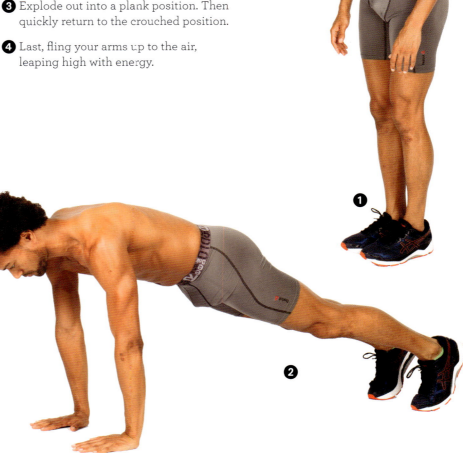

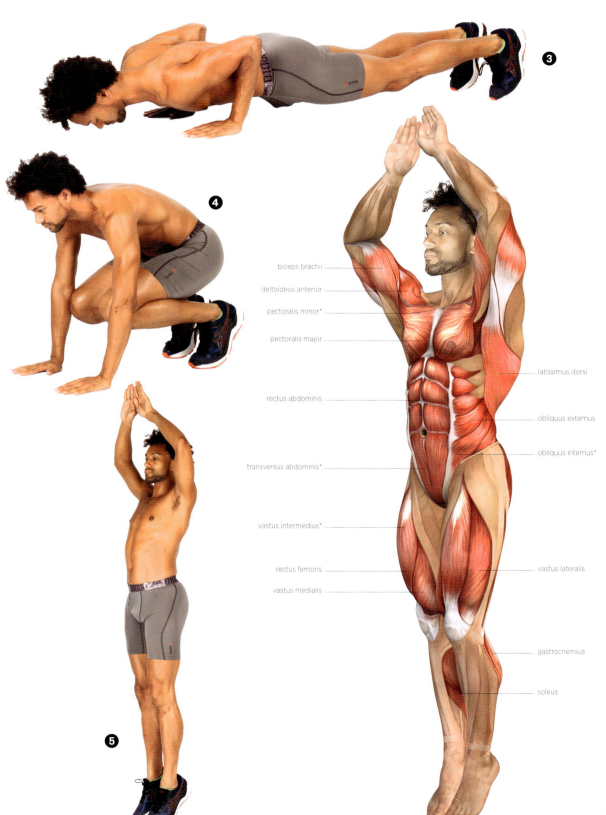

❸

❹

biceps brachii

deltoideus anterior

pectoralis minor*

pectoralis major

latissimus dorsi

rectus abdominis

obliquus externus

obliquus internus*

transversus abdominis*

vastus intermedius*

vastus lateralis

rectus femoris

vastus medialis

gastrocnemius

soleus

❺

WORKOUTS

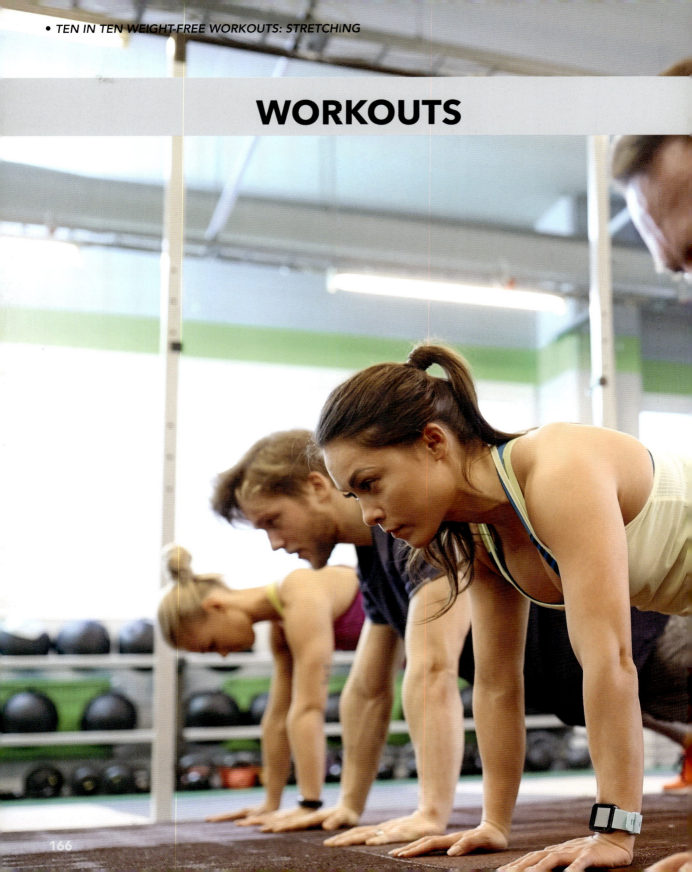

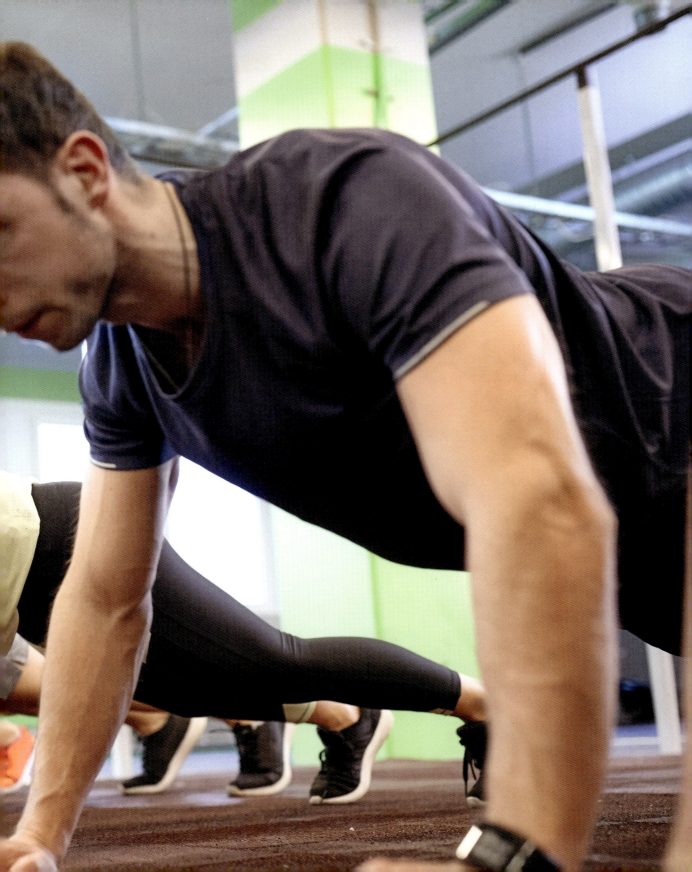

WORKOUTS
THE BASICS

10 min

WARM UP

Jump Rope p58

Half Straddle Stretch p24

Biceps and Pecs Stretch p39

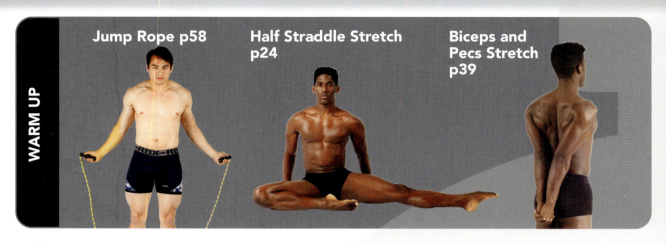

1 Forearm Plank p149

1 MIN TARGETS

BEGINNER
3 x 15 sec holds

INTERMEDIATE
4 x 20 sec holds

ADVANCED
2 x 2 min sec holds

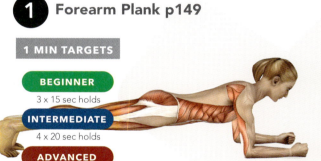

2 Fire Hydrant p72

1 MIN TARGETS

BEGINNER
4 x 10 sec holds + rest

INTERMEDIATE
3 x 15 sec holds + rest

ADVANCED
2 x 30 sec holds

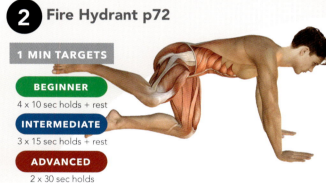

3 Double-Leg Ab Press p94

1 MIN TARGETS

BEGINNER
5 x 10-sec reps

INTERMEDIATE
5 x 15-sec reps

ADVANCED
6 x 20-sec reps

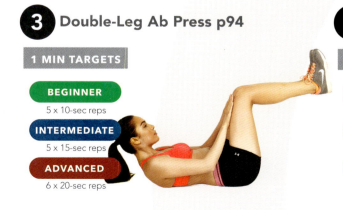

4 Squat p44

1 MIN TARGETS

BEGINNER
4 x 10 sec holds + rest

INTERMEDIATE
4 x 15 sec holds

ADVANCED
3 x 30 sec holds

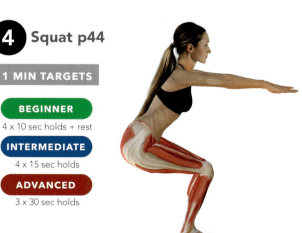

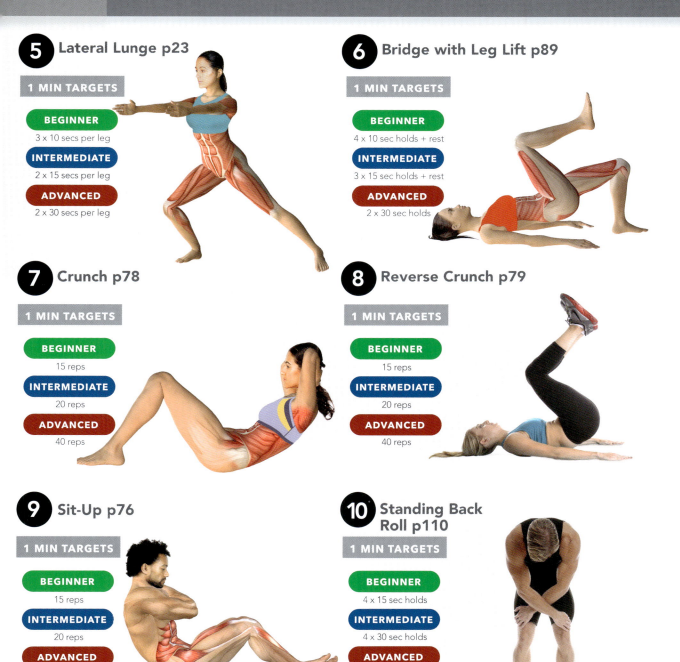

5 Lateral Lunge p23

1 MIN TARGETS

BEGINNER
3 x 10 secs per leg

INTERMEDIATE
2 x 15 secs per leg

ADVANCED
2 x 30 secs per leg

6 Bridge with Leg Lift p89

1 MIN TARGETS

BEGINNER
4 x 10 sec holds + rest

INTERMEDIATE
3 x 15 sec holds + rest

ADVANCED
2 x 30 sec holds

7 Crunch p78

1 MIN TARGETS

BEGINNER
15 reps

INTERMEDIATE
20 reps

ADVANCED
40 reps

8 Reverse Crunch p79

1 MIN TARGETS

BEGINNER
15 reps

INTERMEDIATE
20 reps

ADVANCED
40 reps

9 Sit-Up p76

1 MIN TARGETS

BEGINNER
15 reps

INTERMEDIATE
20 reps

ADVANCED
40 reps

10 Standing Back Roll p110

1 MIN TARGETS

BEGINNER
4 x 15 sec holds

INTERMEDIATE
4 x 30 sec holds

ADVANCED
6 x 30 sec holds

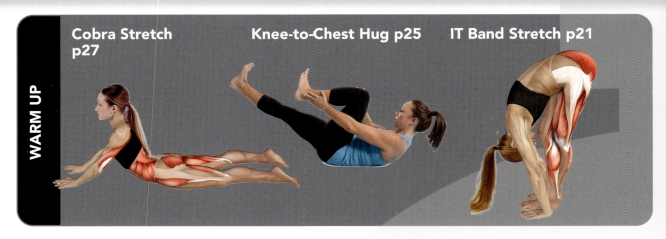

WARM UP

Cobra Stretch p27

Knee-to-Chest Hug p25

IT Band Stretch p21

1 Bicycle Crunch p81

1 MIN TARGETS

BEGINNER
20 kicks

INTERMEDIATE
30 kicks

ADVANCED
50 kicks

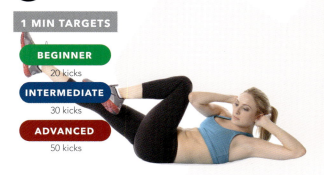

2 Rollover p160

1 MIN TARGETS

BEGINNER
4 x 10 sec holds

INTERMEDIATE
4 x 20 sec holds

ADVANCED
2 x 2 min sec holds

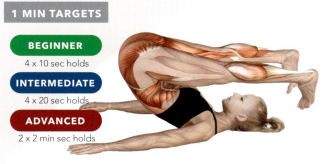

3 Foam Roller Triceps Rollout p163

1 MIN TARGETS

BEGINNER
2 sets 8 reps

INTERMEDIATE
2 sets 15 reps

ADVANCED
30 reps

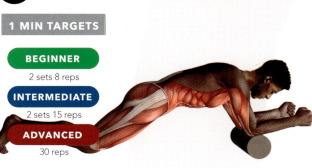

4 Raised-Leg Pike p85

1 MIN TARGETS

BEGINNER
4 x 10 sec holds + rest

INTERMEDIATE
3 x 15 sec holds + rest

ADVANCED
2 x 30 sec holds

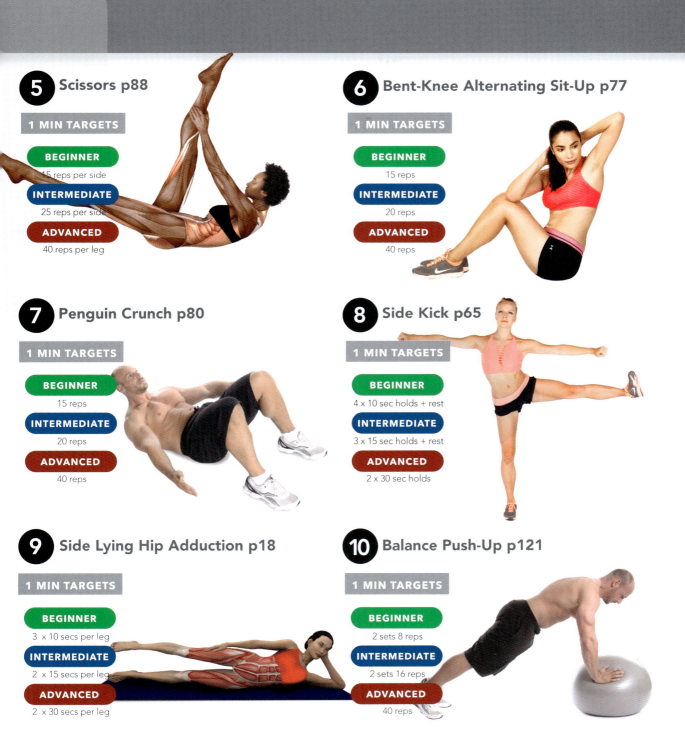

5 Scissors p88

1 MIN TARGETS

BEGINNER
15 reps per side

INTERMEDIATE
25 reps per side

ADVANCED
40 reps per leg

6 Bent-Knee Alternating Sit-Up p77

1 MIN TARGETS

BEGINNER
15 reps

INTERMEDIATE
20 reps

ADVANCED
40 reps

7 Penguin Crunch p80

1 MIN TARGETS

BEGINNER
15 reps

INTERMEDIATE
20 reps

ADVANCED
40 reps

8 Side Kick p65

1 MIN TARGETS

BEGINNER
4 x 10 sec holds + rest

INTERMEDIATE
3 x 15 sec holds + rest

ADVANCED
2 x 30 sec holds

9 Side Lying Hip Adduction p18

1 MIN TARGETS

BEGINNER
3 x 10 secs per leg

INTERMEDIATE
2 x 15 secs per leg

ADVANCED
2 x 30 secs per leg

10 Balance Push-Up p121

1 MIN TARGETS

BEGINNER
2 sets 8 reps

INTERMEDIATE
2 sets 16 reps

ADVANCED
40 reps

WORKOUTS
UPPER ABS

10 min

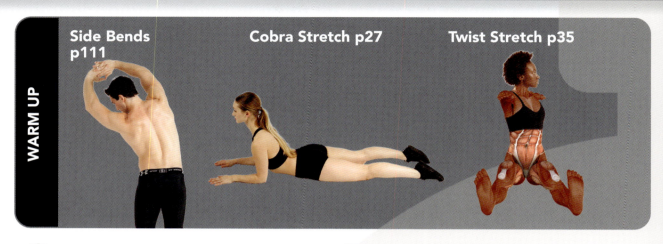

WARM UP

Side Bends p111

Cobra Stretch p27

Twist Stretch p35

1 Alternating Crunch p90

1 MIN TARGETS

BEGINNER
15 reps

INTERMEDIATE
20 reps

ADVANCED
40 reps

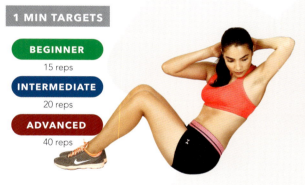

2 Abdominal Kick p87

1 MIN TARGETS

BEGINNER
20 reps per side

INTERMEDIATE
30 reps per side

ADVANCED
50 reps per side

3 Single-Leg V-Up p84

1 MIN TARGETS

BEGINNER
6 reps, 5 sec hold

INTERMEDIATE
10 reps, 5 sec hold

ADVANCED
20 reps, 5 sec hold

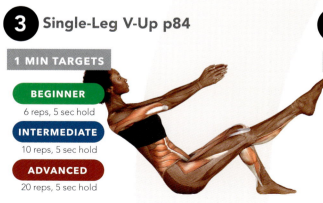

4 Vertical Leg Crunch p82

1 MIN TARGETS

BEGINNER
15 reps

INTERMEDIATE
20 reps

ADVANCED
40 reps

5 V-Up p83

1 MIN TARGETS

BEGINNER
6 reps, 5 sec hold

INTERMEDIATE
10 reps, 5 sec hold

ADVANCED
20 reps, 5 sec hold

6 Back Burner p108

1 MIN TARGETS

BEGINNER
5 x 10-sec sets

INTERMEDIATE
5 x 15-sec sets

ADVANCED
6 x 20-sec sets

7 Swimming p100-1

1 MIN TARGETS

BEGINNER
4 x 10 sec holds + rest

INTERMEDIATE
3 x 15 sec holds + rest

ADVANCED
2 x 30 sec holds

8 Bear Crawl p143

1 MIN TARGETS

BEGINNER
Perform for 1 min

INTERMEDIATE
Perform for 2 mins

ADVANCED
Perform for 3 mins

9 T-Stabilization p159

1 MIN TARGETS

BEGINNER
4 x 10 sec holds

INTERMEDIATE
4 x 20 sec holds

ADVANCED
2 x 2 min sec holds

10 Jackknife p152

1 MIN TARGETS

BEGINNER
3 x 15 sec holds

INTERMEDIATE
4 x 20 sec holds

ADVANCED
2 x 2 min sec holds

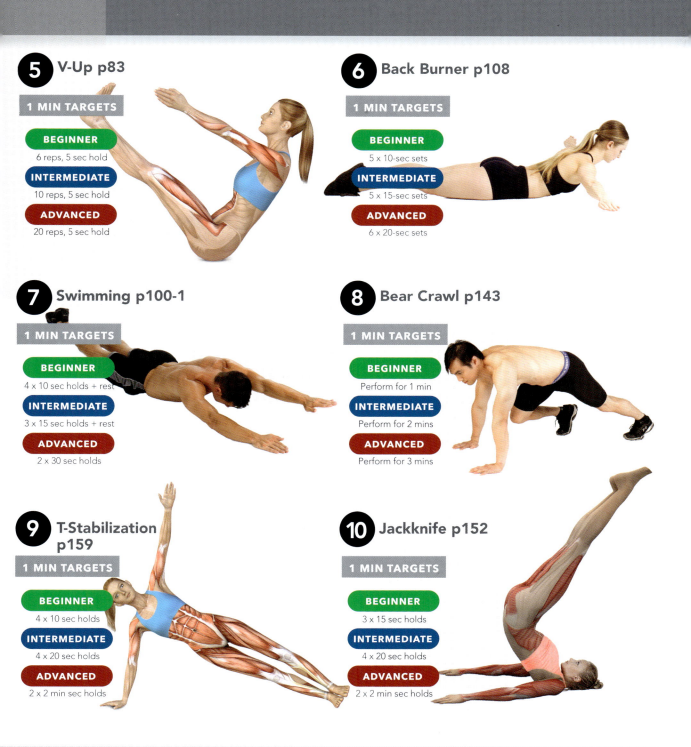

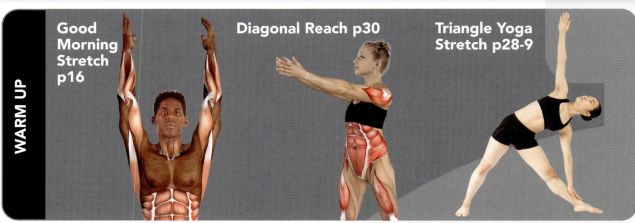

WARM UP

Good Morning Stretch p16

Diagonal Reach p30

Triangle Yoga Stretch p28-9

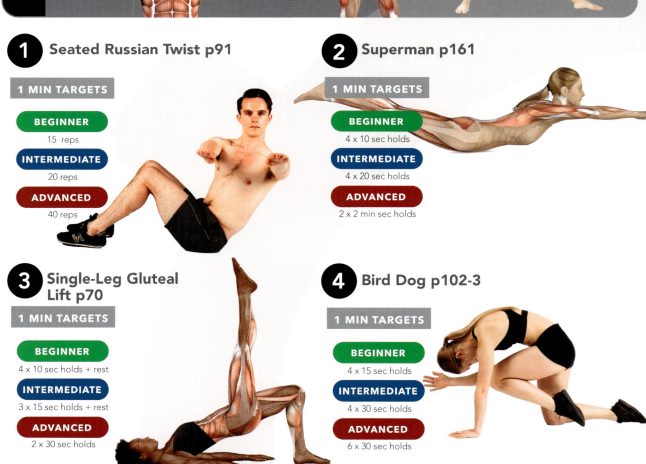

1 Seated Russian Twist p91

1 MIN TARGETS

BEGINNER
15 reps

INTERMEDIATE
20 reps

ADVANCED
40 reps

2 Superman p161

1 MIN TARGETS

BEGINNER
4 x 10 sec holds

INTERMEDIATE
4 x 20 sec holds

ADVANCED
2 x 2 min sec holds

3 Single-Leg Gluteal Lift p70

1 MIN TARGETS

BEGINNER
4 x 10 sec holds + rest

INTERMEDIATE
3 x 15 sec holds + rest

ADVANCED
2 x 30 sec holds

4 Bird Dog p102-3

1 MIN TARGETS

BEGINNER
4 x 15 sec holds

INTERMEDIATE
4 x 30 sec holds

ADVANCED
6 x 30 sec holds

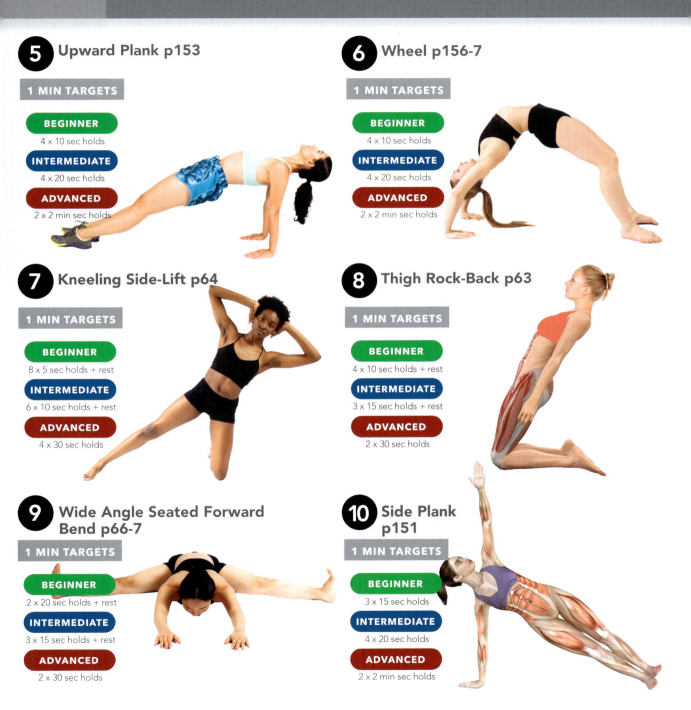

5 Upward Plank p153

1 MIN TARGETS

BEGINNER
4 x 10 sec holds

INTERMEDIATE
4 x 20 sec holds

ADVANCED
2 x 2 min sec holds

6 Wheel p156-7

1 MIN TARGETS

BEGINNER
4 x 10 sec holds

INTERMEDIATE
4 x 20 sec holds

ADVANCED
2 x 2 min sec holds

7 Kneeling Side-Lift p64

1 MIN TARGETS

BEGINNER
8 x 5 sec holds + rest

INTERMEDIATE
6 x 10 sec holds + rest

ADVANCED
4 x 30 sec holds

8 Thigh Rock-Back p63

1 MIN TARGETS

BEGINNER
4 x 10 sec holds + rest

INTERMEDIATE
3 x 15 sec holds + rest

ADVANCED
2 x 30 sec holds

9 Wide Angle Seated Forward Bend p66-7

1 MIN TARGETS

BEGINNER
2 x 20 sec holds + rest

INTERMEDIATE
3 x 15 sec holds + rest

ADVANCED
2 x 30 sec holds

10 Side Plank p151

1 MIN TARGETS

BEGINNER
3 x 15 sec holds

INTERMEDIATE
4 x 20 sec holds

ADVANCED
2 x 2 min sec holds

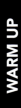 **WORKOUTS**
LEGS

WARM UP

Standing Hamstrings Stretch p17

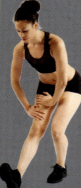

Heel-Drop/ Toe-up Stretch p19

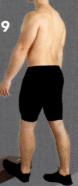

Standing Quad Stretch p22

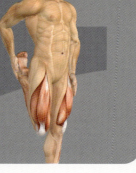

1 Butt Kick p55

1 MIN TARGETS

BEGINNER
Jog in place, 1 min

INTERMEDIATE
Jog in place, 90 secs

ADVANCED
Jog in place, 2 mins

2 Extension Heel Beats p73

1 MIN TARGETS

BEGINNER
4 x 10 beats + rest

INTERMEDIATE
3 x 20 beats

ADVANCED
2 x 30 beats

3 Lateral Step-over p57

1 MIN TARGETS

BEGINNER
20 reps per side

INTERMEDIATE
30 reps per side

ADVANCED
50 reps per leg

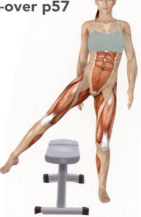

4 One-Legged Bridge p62

1 MIN TARGETS

BEGINNER
4 x 10 sec holds + rest

INTERMEDIATE
3 x 15 sec holds + rest

ADVANCED
2 x 30 sec holds

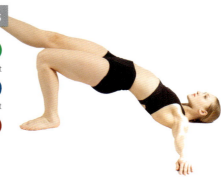

5 High Knees p56

1 MIN TARGETS

BEGINNER
Jog in place, 1 min

INTERMEDIATE
Jog in place, 90 secs

ADVANCED
Jog in place, 2 mins

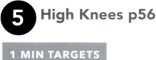
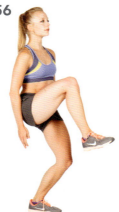

6 Lunge p47

1 MIN TARGETS

BEGINNER
3 x 10 secs per leg

INTERMEDIATE
2 x 15 secs per leg

ADVANCED
2 x 30 secs per leg

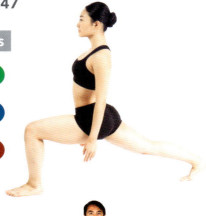

7 Reverse Lunge p50

1 MIN TARGETS

BEGINNER
3 x 10 secs per leg

INTERMEDIATE
2 x 15 secs per leg

ADVANCED
2 x 30 secs per leg

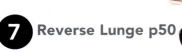
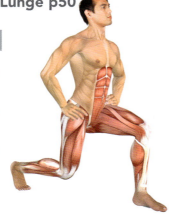

8 Step-Up p60

1 MIN TARGETS

BEGINNER
15 reps per side

INTERMEDIATE
20 reps per side

ADVANCED
30 reps per leg

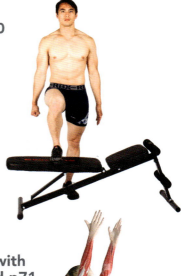

9 Toe Touches p54

1 MIN TARGETS

BEGINNER
8 reps, 5-sec hold

INTERMEDIATE
8 reps, 10 secs per leg

ADVANCED
15 reps, 10 secs per leg

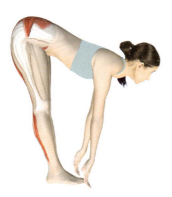

10 Half Squat with Arms Raised p71

1 MIN TARGETS

BEGINNER
4 x 10 sec holds + rest

INTERMEDIATE
4 x 15 sec holds

ADVANCED
3 x 30 sec holds

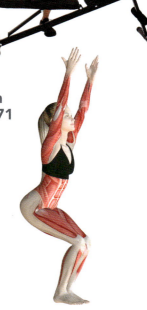

WORKOUTS
CHEST

10 min

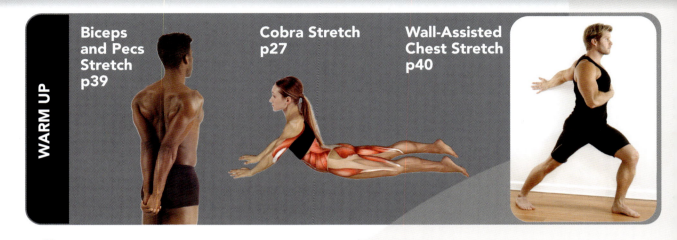

WARM UP

Biceps and Pecs Stretch p39

Cobra Stretch p27

Wall-Assisted Chest Stretch p40

1 Push-Up p114

1 MIN TARGETS

BEGINNER
2 sets 8 reps

INTERMEDIATE
2 sets 16 reps

ADVANCED
40 reps

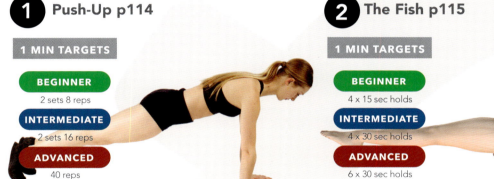

2 The Fish p115

1 MIN TARGETS

BEGINNER
4 x 15 sec holds

INTERMEDIATE
4 x 30 sec holds

ADVANCED
6 x 30 sec holds

3 The Bow p118-9

1 MIN TARGETS

BEGINNER
4 x 10 sec holds + rest

INTERMEDIATE
3 x 15 sec holds + rest

ADVANCED
2 x 30 sec holds

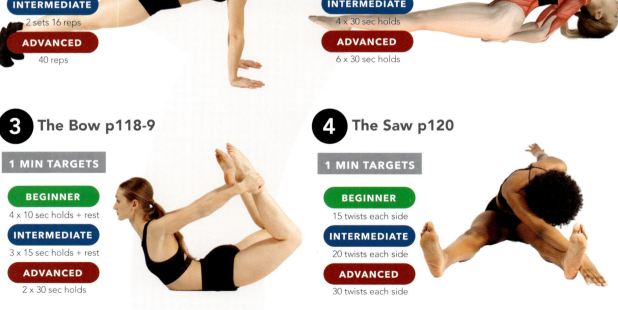

4 The Saw p120

1 MIN TARGETS

BEGINNER
15 twists each side

INTERMEDIATE
20 twists each side

ADVANCED
30 twists each side

5 Towel Fly p123

1 MIN TARGETS

BEGINNER

Perform 3 sets of 8

INTERMEDIATE

Perform 5 sets 8

ADVANCED

Perform 10 sets of 8

6 Plank-Up p124

1 MIN TARGETS

BEGINNER

8 reps

INTERMEDIATE

12 reps

ADVANCED

20 reps

7 Chair Ab Crunch p95

1 MIN TARGETS

BEGINNER

15 reps

INTERMEDIATE

20 reps

ADVANCED

40 reps

8 Plank p148

1 MIN TARGETS

BEGINNER

3 x 15 sec holds

INTERMEDIATE

4 x 20 sec holds

ADVANCED

2 x 2 min sec holds

9 Arm-Reach Plank p150

1 MIN TARGETS

BEGINNER

3 x 15 sec holds

INTERMEDIATE

4 x 20 sec holds

ADVANCED

2 x 2 min sec holds

10 Triceps Push-Up p116-7

1 MIN TARGETS

BEGINNER

2 sets 8 reps

INTERMEDIATE

2 sets 15 reps

ADVANCED

30 reps

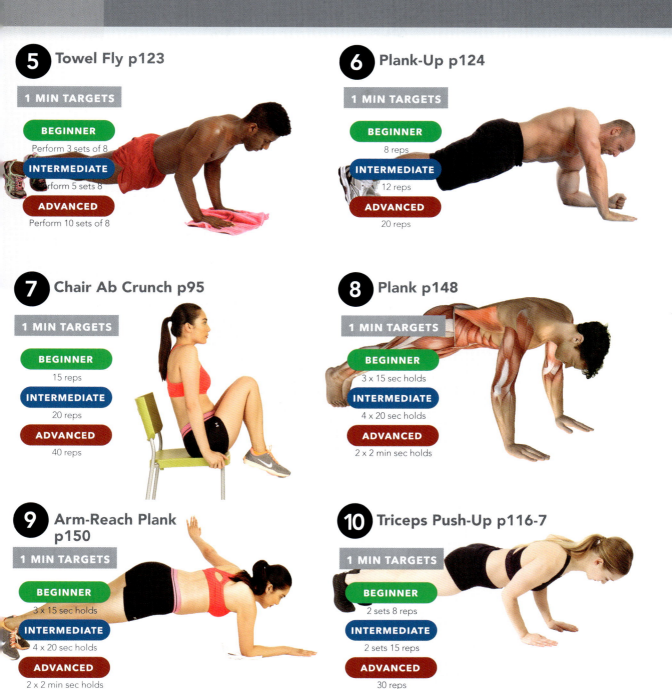

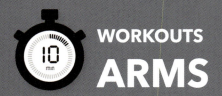

WORKOUTS
ARMS

WARM UP

Good Morning Stretch p16

Shrug p26

Triceps Stretch p38

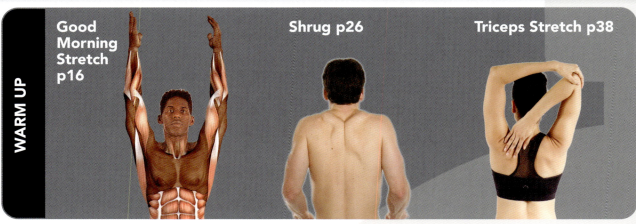

1 Bench Dip p128

1 MIN TARGETS

BEGINNER
4 reps

INTERMEDIATE
6-8 reps

ADVANCED
10+ reps

2 Triceps Dip p129

1 MIN TARGETS

BEGINNER
4 reps

INTERMEDIATE
6-8 reps

ADVANCED
10+ reps

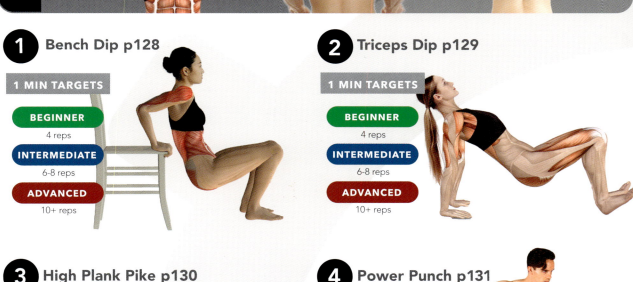

3 High Plank Pike p130

1 MIN TARGETS

BEGINNER
2 x 25 sec holds

INTERMEDIATE
2 x 60 sec holds

ADVANCED
Hold 3 mins

4 Power Punch p131

1 MIN TARGETS

BEGINNER
30 secs each side

INTERMEDIATE
60 secs each side

ADVANCED
2 mins each side

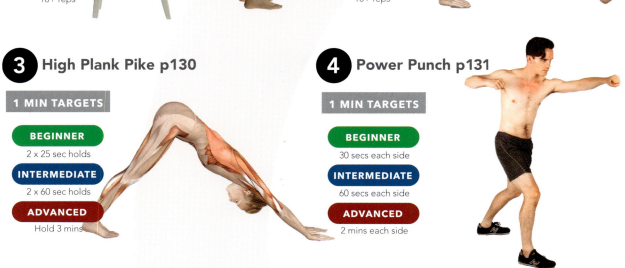

5 Inchworm p132-3

1 MIN TARGETS

BEGINNER
Perform 2 reps

INTERMEDIATE
Perform 4 reps

ADVANCED
Perform 8 reps

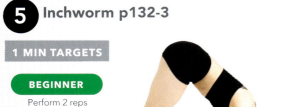

6 Lifting Up p134

1 MIN TARGETS

BEGINNER
4 x 5 sec holds

INTERMEDIATE
4 x 10 sec holds

ADVANCED
4 x 20 sec holds

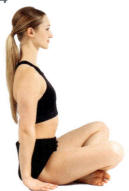

7 Prone Trunk Raise p135

1 MIN TARGETS

BEGINNER
2 x 25 sec holds

INTERMEDIATE
2 x 60 sec holds

ADVANCED
Hold 3 mins

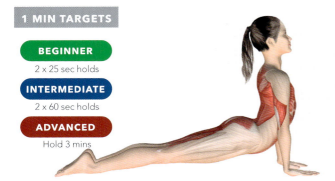

8 Downward Facing Dog p138

1 MIN TARGETS

BEGINNER
2 x 25 sec holds

INTERMEDIATE
2 x 60 sec holds

ADVANCED
Hold 3 mins

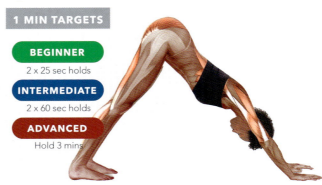

9 Crow p136-7

1 MIN TARGETS

BEGINNER
1 rep, hold 5 secs

INTERMEDIATE
2 reps, hold 10 secs

ADVANCED
2 reps, hold 20 secs

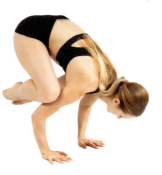

10 Locust p139

1 MIN TARGETS

BEGINNER
4 x 5 sec holds

INTERMEDIATE
4 x 10 sec holds

ADVANCED
4 x 20 sec holds

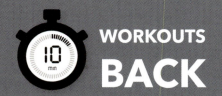

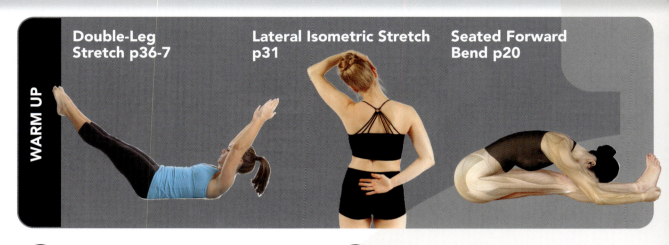

WARM UP

Double-Leg Stretch p36-7

Lateral Isometric Stretch p31

Seated Forward Bend p20

1 Arm-Leg Extension p98

1 MIN TARGETS

BEGINNER
4 x 10 sec holds + rest

INTERMEDIATE
3 x 15 sec holds + rest

ADVANCED
2 x 30 sec holds

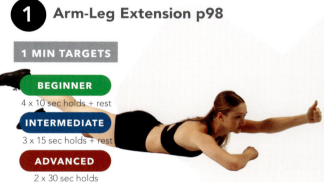

2 Chair twist p106

1 MIN TARGETS

BEGINNER
4 x 15 sec holds

INTERMEDIATE
4 x 30 sec holds

ADVANCED
6 x 30 sec holds

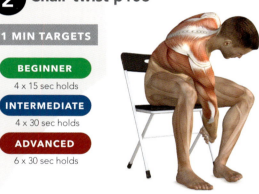

3 Breast Stroke p107

1 MIN TARGETS

BEGINNER
20 reps

INTERMEDIATE
30 reps

ADVANCED
40 reps

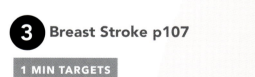

4 Swimming p100-1

1 MIN TARGETS

BEGINNER
4 x 10 sec holds + rest

INTERMEDIATE
3 x 15 sec holds + rest

ADVANCED
2 x 30 sec holds

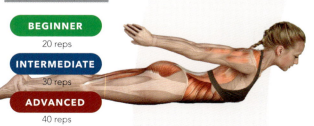

5 Alligator Crawl p144

1 MIN TARGETS

BEGINNER
Perform for 1 min

INTERMEDIATE
Perform for 2 mins

ADVANCED
Perform for 3 mins

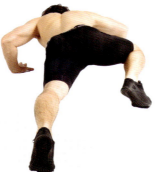

6 Back Burner p108

1 MIN TARGETS

BEGINNER
5 x 10-sec sets

INTERMEDIATE
5 x 15-sec sets

ADVANCED
6 x 20-sec sets

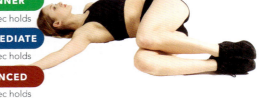

7 Spine Twist p109

1 MIN TARGETS

BEGINNER
15 twists each side

INTERMEDIATE
20 twists each side

ADVANCED
30 twists each side

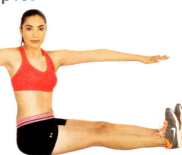

8 Hip Crossover p99

1 MIN TARGETS

BEGINNER
4 x 15 sec holds

INTERMEDIATE
4 x 30 sec holds

ADVANCED
6 x 30 sec holds

9 Side Bends p111

1 MIN TARGETS

BEGINNER
15 bends each side

INTERMEDIATE
15 bends each side

ADVANCED
30 bends each side

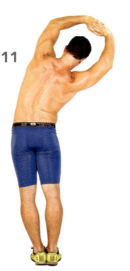

10 Bridge p61

1 MIN TARGETS

BEGINNER
4 x 10 sec holds + rest

INTERMEDIATE
3 x 15 sec holds + rest

ADVANCED
2 x 30 sec holds

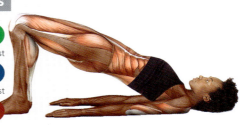

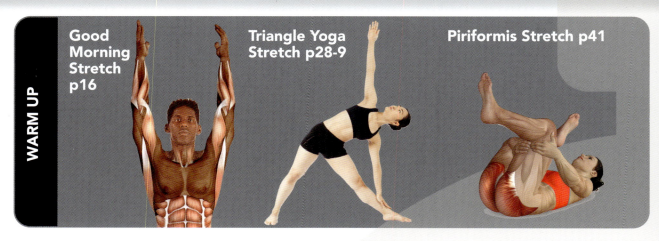

WARM UP

Good Morning Stretch p16

Triangle Yoga Stretch p28-9

Piriformis Stretch p41

1 Deep Lunge p48

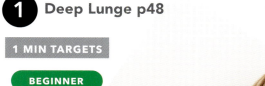

1 MIN TARGETS

BEGINNER
3 x 10 secs per leg

INTERMEDIATE
2 x 15 secs per leg

ADVANCED
2 x 30 secs per leg

2 Swiss Ball Prone Row p92-3

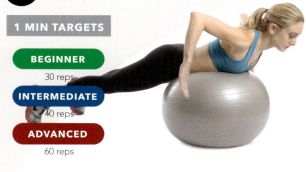

1 MIN TARGETS

BEGINNER
30 reps

INTERMEDIATE
40 reps

ADVANCED
60 reps

3 Swiss Ball Walkaround p122

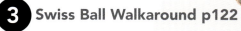

1 MIN TARGETS

BEGINNER
Perform 3 sets

INTERMEDIATE
Perform 5 sets

ADVANCED
Perform 10 sets

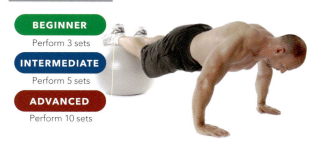

4 Swiss Ball Rollout p125

1 MIN TARGETS

BEGINNER
Perform 8reps

INTERMEDIATE
Perform 15 reps

ADVANCED
Perform 25 reps

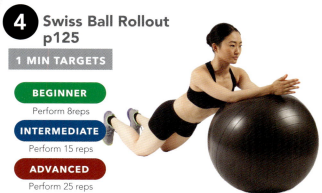

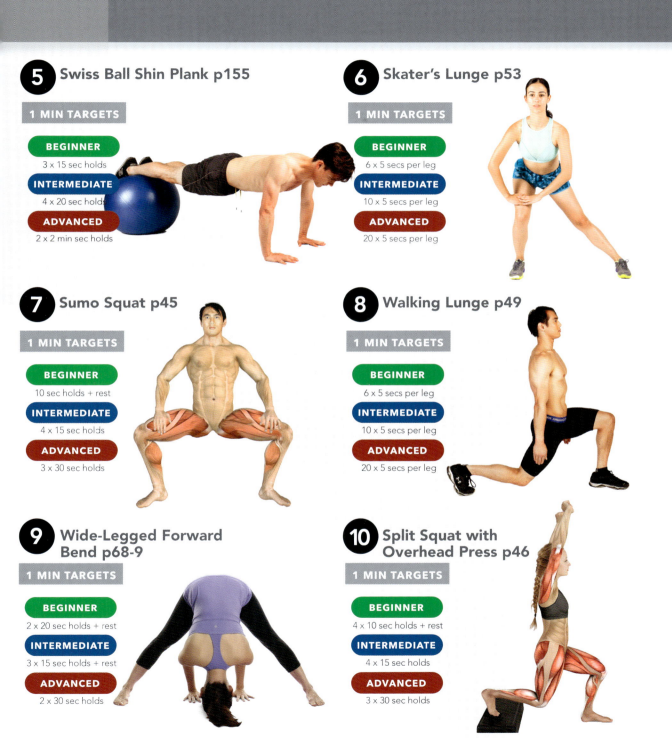

5 Swiss Ball Shin Plank p155

1 MIN TARGETS

BEGINNER
3 x 15 sec holds

INTERMEDIATE
4 x 20 sec holds

ADVANCED
2 x 2 min sec holds

6 Skater's Lunge p53

1 MIN TARGETS

BEGINNER
6 x 5 secs per leg

INTERMEDIATE
10 x 5 secs per leg

ADVANCED
20 x 5 secs per leg

7 Sumo Squat p45

1 MIN TARGETS

BEGINNER
10 sec holds + rest

INTERMEDIATE
4 x 15 sec holds

ADVANCED
3 x 30 sec holds

8 Walking Lunge p49

1 MIN TARGETS

BEGINNER
6 x 5 secs per leg

INTERMEDIATE
10 x 5 secs per leg

ADVANCED
20 x 5 secs per leg

9 Wide-Legged Forward Bend p68-9

1 MIN TARGETS

BEGINNER
2 x 20 sec holds + rest

INTERMEDIATE
3 x 15 sec holds + rest

ADVANCED
2 x 30 sec holds

10 Split Squat with Overhead Press p46

1 MIN TARGETS

BEGINNER
4 x 10 sec holds + rest

INTERMEDIATE
4 x 15 sec holds

ADVANCED
3 x 30 sec holds

WORKOUTS
TOTAL BODY

10 min

WARM UP

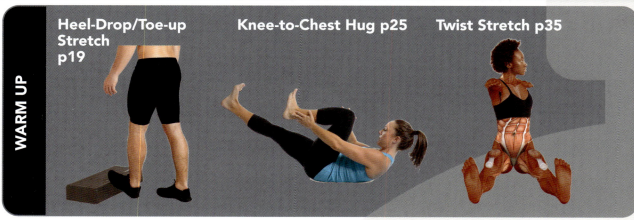

Heel-Drop/Toe-up Stretch p19

Knee-to-Chest Hug p25

Twist Stretch p35

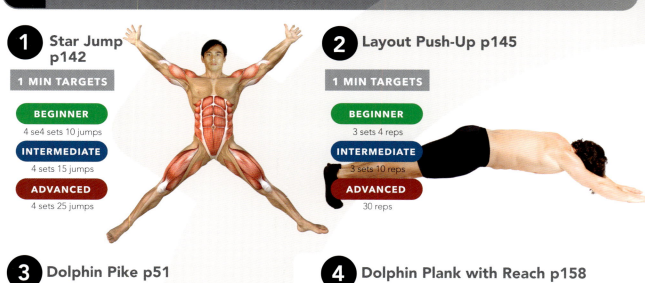

1 Star Jump p142

1 MIN TARGETS

BEGINNER
4 se4 sets 10 jumps

INTERMEDIATE
4 sets 15 jumps

ADVANCED
4 sets 25 jumps

2 Layout Push-Up p145

1 MIN TARGETS

BEGINNER
3 sets 4 reps

INTERMEDIATE
3 sets 10 reps

ADVANCED
30 reps

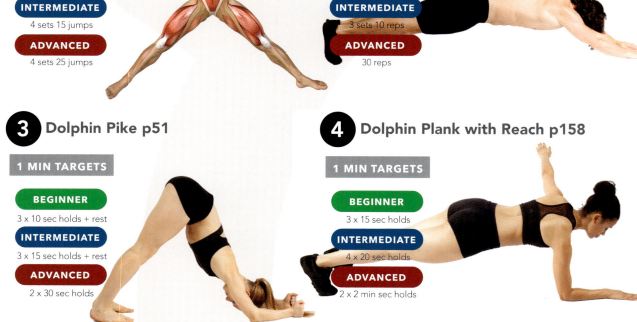

3 Dolphin Pike p51

1 MIN TARGETS

BEGINNER
3 x 10 sec holds + rest

INTERMEDIATE
3 x 15 sec holds + rest

ADVANCED
2 x 30 sec holds

4 Dolphin Plank with Reach p158

1 MIN TARGETS

BEGINNER
3 x 15 sec holds

INTERMEDIATE
4 x 20 sec holds

ADVANCED
2 x 2 min sec holds

5 Frog Straddle p59

1 MIN TARGETS

BEGINNER
4 x 10 sec holds + rest

INTERMEDIATE
3 x 15 sec holds + rest

ADVANCED
2 x 30 sec holds

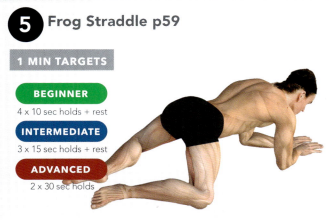

6 Lateral Extension Reverse Lunge p52

1 MIN TARGETS

BEGINNER
3 x 10 secs per leg

INTERMEDIATE
2 x 15 secs per leg

ADVANCED
2 x 30 secs per leg

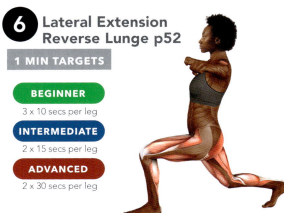

7 Chaturanga Plank p154

1 MIN TARGETS

BEGINNER
3 x 15 sec holds

INTERMEDIATE
4 x 20 sec holds

ADVANCED
2 x 2 min sec holds

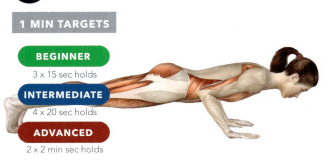

8 Tabletop March p162

1 MIN TARGETS

BEGINNER
3 x 15 sec holds

INTERMEDIATE
4 x 20 sec holds

ADVANCED
2 x 2 min sec holds

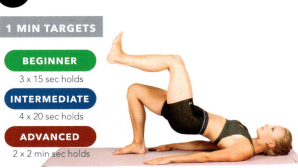

9 Turkish Get-Up p146

1 MIN TARGETS

BEGINNER
4 reps

INTERMEDIATE
8 reps

ADVANCED
15 reps

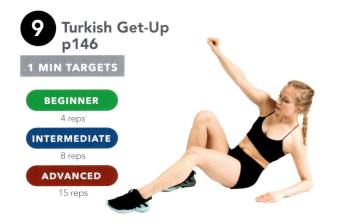

10 Burpee p164-5

1 MIN TARGETS

BEGINNER
4 reps

INTERMEDIATE
8 reps

ADVANCED
15 reps

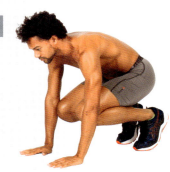

ICON INDEX

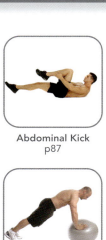
Abdominal Kick
p87

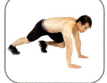
Alligator Crawl
p144

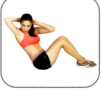
Alternating Crunch
p90

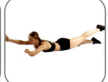
Arm-Leg Extension
p98

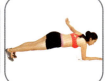
Arm-Reach Plank
p150

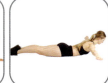
Back Burner
p108

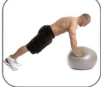
Balance Push-Up
p121

Bear Crawl
p143

Bench Dip
p128

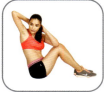
Bent-Knee
Alternating Sit-Up
p77

Biceps and Pecs
Stretch
p39

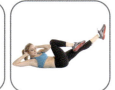
Bicycle Crunch
p81

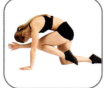
Bird Dog
p102-3

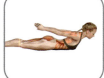
Breast Stroke
p86-7

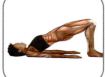
Bridge
p61

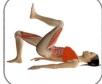
Bridge with Leg Lift
p89

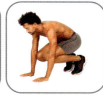
Burpee
p164-5

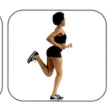
Butt Kick
p55

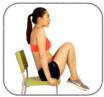
Chair Ab Crunch
p95

Chair Twist
p106

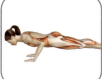
Chaturanga Plank
p154

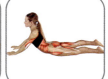
Cobra Stretch
p27

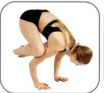
Crow
p136-7

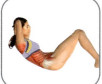
Crunch
p78

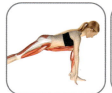
Deep Lunge
p48

Diagonal Reach
p30

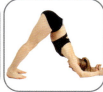
Dolphin Pike
p51

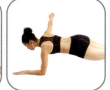
Dolphin Plank with
Reach
p158

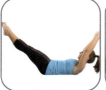
Double-Leg Stretch
p36-7

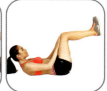
Double-Leg Ab Press
p94

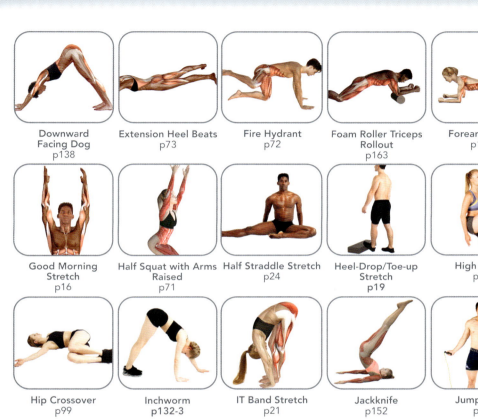

Downward Facing Dog p138

Extension Heel Beats p73

Fire Hydrant p72

Foam Roller Triceps Rollout p163

Forearm Plank p149

Frog Straddle p59

Good Morning Stretch p16

Half Squat with Arms Raised p71

Half Straddle Stretch p24

Heel-Drop/Toe-up Stretch p19

High Knees p56

High Plank Pike p130

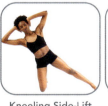 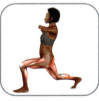 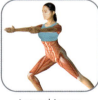 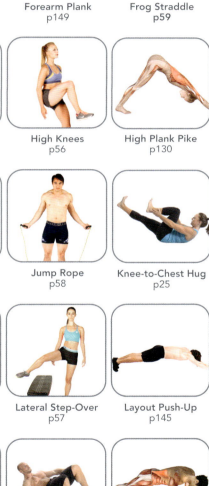 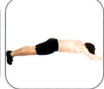

Hip Crossover p99

Inchworm p132-3

IT Band Stretch p21

Jackknife p152

Jump Rope p58

Knee-to-Chest Hug p25

Kneeling Side-Lift p64

Lateral Extension Reverse Lunge p52

Lateral Isometric Stretch p31

Lateral Lunge p23

Lateral Step-Over p57

Layout Push-Up p145

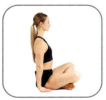 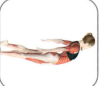 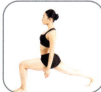 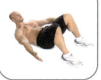 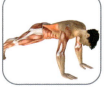

Lifting Up p134

Locust p139

Lunge p47

One-Legged Bridge p62

Penguin Crunch p80

Plank p148

ICON INDEX

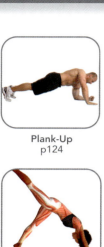
Plank-Up
p124

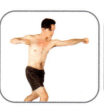
Power Punch
p131

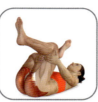
Piriformis Stretch
p41

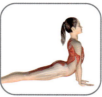
Prone Trunk Raise
p135

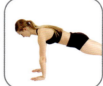
Push-Up
p114

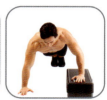
Push-Up Hand
Walk-Over
p120

Raised-Leg pike
p85

Reverse Crunch
p79

Reverse Lunge
p50

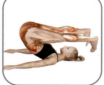
Rollover
p160

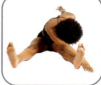
Saw Stretch
p34-5

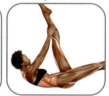
Scissors
p88

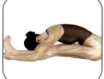
Seated Forward
Bend
p20

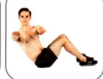
Seated Russian Twist
p91

Shrug
p26

Side Bends
p111

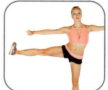
Side Kick
p65

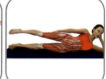
Side Lying Hip
Adduction
p18

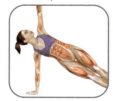
Side Plank
p151

Single-Leg
Gluteal Lift
p70

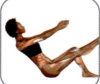
Single-Leg V-Up
p84

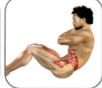
Sit-Up
p76

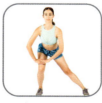
Skater's Lunge
p53

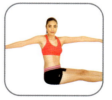
Spine Twist
p109

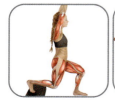
Split Squat with
Overhead Press
p46

Squat
p44

Standing Back Roll
p110

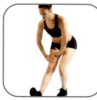
Standing Hamstrings
Stretch
p17

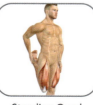
Standing Quad
Stretch
p22

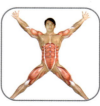
Star Jump
p142

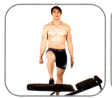
Step-Up
p60

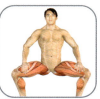
Sumo Squat
p45

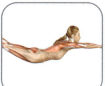
Superman
p161

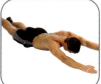
Swimming
p100-1

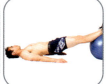
Swiss Ball Bridge
p86

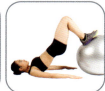
Swiss Ball
Hamstrings Curl
p32-3

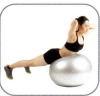
Swiss Ball
Hyperextension
p104-5

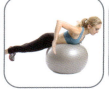
Swiss Ball Prone Row
p92-3

Swiss Ball Rollout
p125

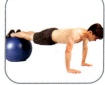
Swiss Ball Shin Plank
p155

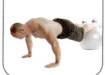
Swiss Ball
Walkaround
p122

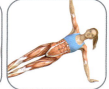
T-Stabilization
p159

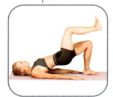
Tabletop March
p182

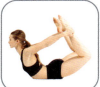
The Bow
p118-9

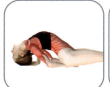
The Fish
p115

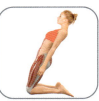
Thigh Rock-Back
p63

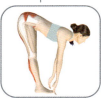
Toe Touches
p54

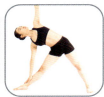
Triangle Yoga Stretch
p28-9

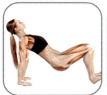
Triceps Dip
p129

Triceps Push-Up
p116-7

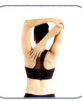
Triceps Stretch
p38

Turkish Get-Up
p146-7

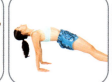
Upward Plank
p153

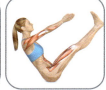
V-Up
p83

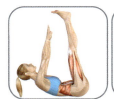
Vertical Leg Crunch
p82

Walking Lunge
p49

Wall-Assisted Chest
Stretch
p40

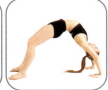
Wheel
p156-7

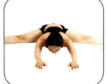
Wide Angle Seated
Forward Bend
p66-7

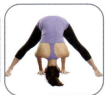
Wide-Legged
Forward Bend
p68-9

CREDITS

All exercise models in this book are from moseleyroad.inc.
For any individual model information, please contact: amoore@moseleyroad.com

All other images are from shuttterstock.
P9 - Lizardflms. P11&166 - Ground Picture. p14 - Rocksweeper. p42 - Ihor Bulyhin. p74 - UfaBizPhoto. p96 - Satyrenko.
p112 - antoniodiaz. p126 - Jacob Lund. p140 - F8 studio.

Special thanks to Dil.